Workouts for Seniors

Simple Home Exercises for Improved Strength, Balance, and Energy

Free Bonuses from Scott Hamrick available for limited time

Hi seniors!

My name is Scott Hamrick, and first off, I want to THANK YOU for reading my book.

Now you have a chance to join my exclusive "workout for seniors" email list so you can get the ebook below for free as well as the potential to get more ebooks for seniors for free! Simply click the link below to join.

P.S. Remember that it's 100% free to join the list.

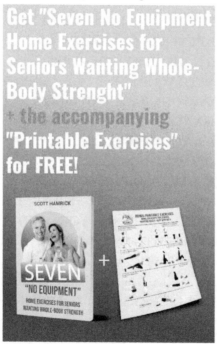

Access your free bonuses here
https://livetolearn.lpages.co/workouts-for-seniors-paperback/

Table of Contents

Introduction

Peter smiled into his glass as his mind returned to just a few years before. He had just recently retired from his job as an accountant with the Ministry of Agriculture. At the time, he was unsure, unhappy, and anxious about his future. Besides, he knew he was out of shape as he just didn't feel good. He had body and joint aches, chronic digestive issues, and trouble remembering little things. He was sure that his body could fail him at any moment.

Now just years later, at 69, Peter felt healthier and more confident than he had in ages. One day, his wife told him, "I saw your sister, Sharon, and she says you must tell her your secret to your reversing aging." Peter was a little startled when he heard that. But then, he laughed and replied, "I don't tell that story for the fun of it. If she's ready to do what I did, then she can come, and I'll tell her. If not..." he shrugged; dismissing the topic and turning his full attention to what he was doing.

Peter was one of those I mentored on how to keep fit and healthy, even as a senior.

I got interested in physical fitness for seniors when I observed that those who lived the longest weren't necessarily those who were financially well-to-do. Any senior who found a way to remain physically active seemed happier and healthier despite their situation. Many of them even lived in villages and still worked on their farms. I realized that the common factor among these successful seniors was that they remained active even as they got older.

You may be getting along in age and feeling anxious about your health. It's natural to be concerned that you may not remain independent and mentally sound as you age.

Research has shown that regular exercise can benefit healthy seniors and older adults with health conditions such as arthritis, high blood pressure, and obesity. If you desire to age gracefully and are interested in taking action in terms of physical fitness *regardless of your age*, this is a book you want to pay attention to!

Included are guidelines, exercise tips, and lifestyle changes to equip and strengthen your body for the years ahead. We've tried to make it as simple to understand and practice as possible. Of course, you must consult your physician before you start any exercise regimen; their guidance will help you ascertain the level of intensity to begin at. While some exercises aren't suitable for those with restrictions, there is always a modification that can be substituted.

We hope that you will not only read through to educate yourself but also help yourself by putting what you read into practice. Be assured that your body will reward you for acting.

Chapter 1 The Benefits of Working Out as a Senior

Senior citizens are encouraged to get at least 2.5 hours of moderate exercise weekly. This may not be easy, though, because you tend to become less energetic and, therefore, less active as you age. These slowdowns are natural and expected as the body undergoes many changes as it ages.

These changes include slower metabolism, stiffening of blood vessels, shrinkage, reduction of bone density, etc. All these changes contribute to making it more challenging to stay active as you get along in age.

Exercise is important for people of all ages. You need to engage in physical activities regardless of age to keep the body and mind active. However, as you approach your golden years, the importance of exercise cannot be overemphasized. Most people believe you should slow down as you age, but that's not entirely true.

While it's true that there are activities that are not recommended for you to participate in (your exercise routines will look different from that of a younger person), it is still very important that you continue to be active.

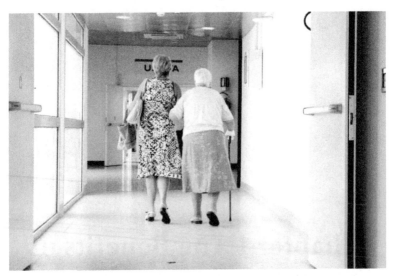

1. An elderly lady supported by a younger woman and a cane.
https://pixabay.com/photos/senior-citizens-aisle-doctor-1461424

It could even be argued that a senior citizen requires exercise more than a younger person to maintain their quality of life. You also need exercise to ensure that you can genuinely enjoy your later years. It doesn't matter whether you had been an athlete or bodybuilder from when you were younger. It also doesn't matter if you've always lived a sedentary lifestyle, as exercise is crucial as you advance in years. Exercising now and continuing to stay active will keep your mind and body happy and healthy for tomorrow.

You can (and should) start exercising, even if you have never done so before. Depending on your present conditioning, you will have to adjust your exercise routine to suit the current state of your body. The theory that you shouldn't exercise or stop exercising as you age is a myth and could prove to be very harmful to you.

To live long and enjoy your life, you must incorporate functional activity into your lifestyle. If you're on the fence about whether to start or continue working out in your old age or not, here are some specific benefits to help you make up your mind.

Benefits of Exercise for an Older Adult

1. It Can Help You Lose Weight, Maintain a Healthy Weight or Build Muscle

Many people wonder if losing weight when you're over sixty is feasible. Not only is it achievable, but you can also *gain muscle*. It's certainly not going to be as easy as it would have been in your 20s or 30s, but it's not impossible either.

Slower metabolism rate and responses to hormonal and neurological impulses are all changes the body begins to undergo as it ages. These changes make weight loss and muscle gain a little more difficult but not impossible. You must, however, be deliberate about your goal.

Losing weight is the same process for you as for a younger person. It would require burning more calories through activity than you consumed. Eating healthy foods without empty or excess calories and exercising regularly will help you lose weight.

The same goes for building muscle - it's the same process for a younger person. When you engage in strength training and weightlifting, it can cause little tears in your muscles. Your body repairs those muscles with protein from your diet, and the muscles become bigger and stronger.

The only difference is that while a younger body can produce new muscles, your body only repairs broken down muscles. The result is not different; however, you would still have bigger and stronger muscles to show for your work. The thought of big muscles may not be ideal for those over a certain age, but it's more likely that much-needed strength and stability will come from weight training long before any obvious muscle size increases.

While gaining muscle or losing weight as an older adult isn't going to be easy (it's a challenge for everyone), the results will undoubtedly be worth the effort with a bit of work and dedication.

2. It Can Help You Feel Younger and Improve your Energy Levels

Many believe you should slow down on physical activities as you age to conserve energy or play it safe. Research shows that the reverse should be the case. Slowing down can be detrimental in the long run. It can make you become sluggish and feel like you have less energy. You may even begin to feel moody and depressed all the time.

Many older people experience a dip in their energy levels and have days in which they just feel sleepy, tired, and lack motivation for anything. When you feel like that, a very good way to shake those feelings is to get yourself up and get moving! Get some exercise by taking a walk around your neighborhood, doing some yoga or stretches, or even dancing.

These activities help to improve blood circulation in the body, getting oxygen and nutrients to flow better. They also result in the release of neurotransmitters such as endorphins. The result of this is an improved mood and regained energy.

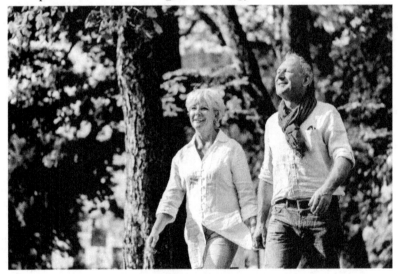
2. Elderly couple walking

3. It Can Reduce the Risk and Symptoms of Chronic Illnesses

Chronic illnesses such as diabetes, high blood pressure, arthritis, and even some cancer can be prevented through exercise. Therefore, the importance of exercise to your overall health can never be overlooked. Regular exercise helps to improve the efficiency of cardiovascular, digestive, and respiratory activities and exercise serves as the fuel to help keep the body running properly.

Even when chronic diseases are already present, the symptoms can be alleviated and kept from getting worse by regular exercise.

In the case of high blood pressure, for example, engaging in moderate aerobics daily can help prevent symptoms and even reduce the risk of dying from heart failure. Cardio helps to improve heart function, which may lower that blood pressure while strengthening the heart muscles.

In type 2 diabetes, regular exercise can make the action of insulin more effective, reducing the effects of negative symptoms, and it can also prevent complications related to diabetes from worsening.

Exercise is beneficial for those with asthma because it can go a long way in preventing the occurrence of crises and reducing their severity by boosting the endurance of the lungs.

In arthritis, back pain, and other conditions affecting body movement, flexibility, and balance, exercise can help you remain mobile, improve stability, and even reduce the occurrence of pain.

It is always necessary to consult with your physician before starting any workout routine; he'll likely have recommendations and precautions for you to follow. He'll be able to advise you on the intensity of exercise your body can withstand and what routines you should avoid.

4. It Can Help You Maintain Your Independence

One of the fears many people have regarding aging is the possibility of losing their independence and having to rely on others for such simple activities as going to the restroom, putting on their clothes, feeding themselves, or even putting on their shoes.

Nobody likes the thought that they would, someday, have to constantly burden others with doing simple things for them. In fact, many people say that they would rather not live to see the day they can no longer take care of themselves.

As grim as this sounds, the good news is that exercise has been shown to help the elderly maintain their independence for a longer time. Research has shown that those who don't exercise in their old age lose a large percentage of muscle mass, and losing muscle mass is synonymous with losing independence.

When you exercise regularly, you make use of your muscles repeatedly. This gives your body the signal that they are still needed; hence your body continues to send nutrients into your various muscles. Muscles allow you to do things like get up from a chair, pick something up off the ground and reach overhead to put something in a kitchen cabinet.

Balance exercises can prevent falls which can become more common as you age. The trouble is that when an elderly person falls, the chances of recovery are slimmer than those ten or fifteen years younger. If there's no recovery, an elderly fall victim can automatically become dependent on others.

Any type of physical activity can help to promote independence in the elderly. It's best to incorporate different kinds of exercises, though. Aerobic exercises are great to help you stay mobile. Strength exercises make it possible for you to lift things (even grandkids); balance exercises help prevent you from

falling while stretching exercises help maintain flexibility for bending and turning.

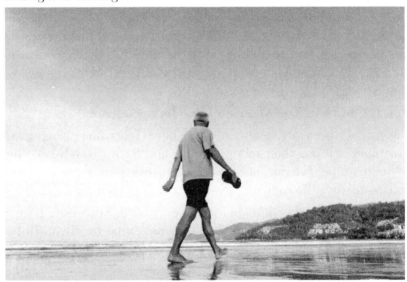

3. A senior walking independently at the beach
https://pixabay.com/photos/beach-senior-man-male-walking-2090091/

5. It helps to Improve Brain Function and Prevent Dementia

In addition to the effects on physical functions, aging also affects mental function. As you age, there can be shrinkage of the frontal lobe and hippocampus (the parts of the brain responsible for multitasking, recall, and attention). There is also a reduction in the production of chemicals that protect the brain, support memory, and aid in effective thinking.

The result of this reduction from aging can lead to cognitive struggles and, in the worst case, conditions such as dementia or Alzheimer's. The prevalence of these conditions, though, also depends on other factors such as genetics, gender, and lifestyle.

Of these factors, the only one that can be effectively controlled is *lifestyle*. Maintaining a healthy lifestyle (by having a nutritious diet, exercising regularly, not smoking, and drinking in moderation or not at all) can reduce an individual's risk of developing conditions like dementia.

However, several studies have shown that physical exercise has a more significant effect on the mental ability of an older adult than any other factor.

More thorough research still needs to be carried out to identify the specific exercises that can be proven to directly prevent dementia. However, the studies that have been carried out show that a combination of aerobics and strength-training exercises helps improve brain function. In one study, it was observed that the size of subjects' hippocampus had increased after a year of regular exercising. That was a reversal of about two years of aging. Imagine being able to get back two years of clarity and memory by simply being active and increasing physical activity!

Even simple physical activities that increase your heart rate, such as brisk walking and jogging for 30 to 60 minutes daily, can improve cognitive activity, reasoning, and memory.

6. It Can Improve the Quality of Your Sleep

It's been said that older adults require less sleep than they did when they were younger, and this is not entirely true as sleep requirements for adults remain constant. However, you may experience a change in your sleeping habits, such as feeling sleepy earlier in the evenings, waking up earlier in the mornings and sleeping lightly, or waking up several times at night.

These are normal changes that occur with age. They can be attributed to several hormonal changes, as the body produces lower quantities of certain hormones such as melatonin, testosterone, and estrogen as it ages. Hormones naturally produced by the body are the reason you feel sleepy at bedtime and rested in the morning. As the body ages, these feelings may shift or lessen because the hormones are not being produced at the same rate anymore.

While all these changes may be considered normal, it is not normal to wake up tired all the time. It's also not normal for you to be unable to fall asleep and stay asleep. These are signs that something needs to be addressed to maintain quality of life. If you're experiencing issues such as these, it's necessary to speak with a physician. They may, in turn, prescribe something to help balance these hormones or even suggest increasing exercise.

Exercising during the day can make you feel more tired towards the end of the day, which is conducive to sleep. The increased blood and oxygen circulation, as well as the release of endorphins brought about by exercise, help increase the feelings of well-being and reduce stress. Less stress can help enhance relaxation at night and support a peaceful mind for sleep. All these factors can be used as part of a routine to contribute to deeper and better sleep.

7. It Can Help You Meet New People and Grow Your Social Circle

Getting older can result in many seniors staying indoors all day, every day. There isn't always a pressing reason to get up and go out; sometimes, it simply feels like a hassle. We already know this doesn't help your physical well-being because activity equals health. However, it doesn't help your social or emotional well-being either. Falling into an emotional rut can have devastating consequences if you're often alone or already dealing with the other challenges of aging.

Not meeting and interacting with people could make you feel demotivated, weak, tired, or even depressed. While you may be retired and no longer have a job that takes you outside daily, you don't have to stay home alone all day.

If you're starting to feel bored, lonely, or even tired during the day, a walk around the neighborhood might be just what you need to get your spirits up. Alternatively, walking over to talk to a neighbor or meeting up with a friend may be activity enough, depending on restrictions. Just seeing a friendly face can do wonders for boosting your mood and provide a source of motivation. You could even take things a step further by joining a gym or a group of older adults who want to stay physically active.

Walk groups or gym buddies can add an additional level of joy and accountability to being active.

Not only would you be doing your body and mind good, but there's also the bonus advantage of meeting and making friends with other seniors who have similar interests as you.

You never know how far these relationships can go. Finding a walking partner or gym buddy could drastically improve your life as a senior. You may enjoy your new acquaintances and socializing so much that you find other fun and interesting activities to do together besides working out!

Who says you shouldn't live a social life because you're getting older? Having a new social circle could do wonders for all aspects of your life while making you feel young again.

Are you excited yet about the prospect of starting an exercise routine? I hope you're convinced by now that not only can you start exercising in your later years, but you should also start immediately. The benefits are endless and backed by years of science and endless testimonials from seniors who've added fitness to their lives.

Staying active is not only likely to help you live longer, but it will keep the senior years more vibrant and meaningful. If you're ready to begin your active, healthy, and graceful aging journey, let this book serve as your guide.

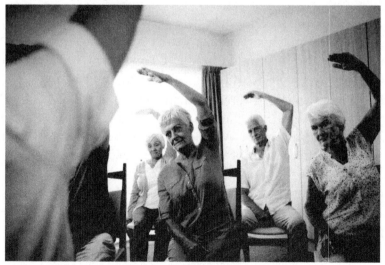

4. Senior citizens exercising in a group.

Chapter 2 When Should I Work Out?

Now that we've established the benefits of exercising as an older adult, it's time to dive into the details and answer all your pressing questions. You're probably wondering how long to exercise, what time to exercise, and how frequently you should exercise, along with a host of other questions.

This chapter will begin to address these questions, starting with when to exercise.

Depending on your lifestyle, you may or may not have a lot of time on your hands or maintain a strict schedule. Your timing for exercise may also be affected by where you choose to exercise, i.e., whether you're exercising at home, at the gym, or in a group.

For younger adults, exercise is beneficial at any time of the day. For the elderly, however, there's a need to put a little more thought into the timing for activity. While some seniors exercise first thing in the morning after a cup of coffee, some wait till the afternoon or early evening to work out. These choices are likely not based on when the best time to work out is but instead on preference.

In other words, those who work out in the mornings probably do so because they are morning people – and that time feels natural for them. Others have more time in the evening or feel more energetic later in the day, hence their choice to work out in the evenings.

It's great to pick an exercise time that you are happy and comfortable with, but there may be optimal times to do it depending on what you hope to gain from your workout.

Before we go into the pros and cons of working out at a specific time in detail, it should be said that most seniors shouldn't work out close to bedtime (3 hours or less). One of the effects of working out is stimulation, and this is not something you want to be happening in your body close to bedtime.

Feeling stimulated and energized at bedtime can significantly affect the quality of your sleep, preventing you from getting the benefits you desired when you started working out in the first place. You'll want to tire yourself out with exercise earlier in the day and relax before bedtime to ensure you get good sleep to help aid your recovery.

The following sections will compare the specific benefits of working out in the morning, afternoon, or evening.

Benefits of Working out in the Morning

1. You Can Be More Productive

Hitting the gym or going for a run early in the morning, as soon as you wake up, can be a great practice that gives you a sense of achievement and pride in yourself. Knowing that you started the day, choosing the path of resistance and discipline can give you a sense of accomplishment.

Having accomplished something so early makes it easier for you to keep going during the day and gives you the momentum to be more productive and stay on track in other important areas of your life. It also helps to check exercise off your list for the day, so the rest of it is free to be filled with other activities.

Exercise is also great for mood, energy, and mental clarity. The increased circulation and release of positive hormones may be just what you need to power you through the rest of the day, like an early extra cup of coffee.

2. There's a Greater Chance of Consistency

A more significant percentage of those who work out do so in the mornings, which seems like the most favorable time for working out. One of the reasons for this is that motivation or willpower is higher in the mornings. Many habitual exercises do their daily workout first thing in the morning. This is because it's easy to become a habit if it's always done first and at the same time. Nothing can get in the way of a workout if it's always the first thing started and completed for the day.

Later in the day, you may feel too tired, eat too big of a lunch, or something may come up that requires your attention elsewhere. Then either the workout gets missed or pushed into possibly affecting sleep if done before bedtime.

The body may also get used to the daily morning boost and become more accustomed to the practice of being physically active first thing. Exercise may eventually become something you and your body look forward to upon waking.

3. It Can Make You Happier or Boost Your Mood for the Rest of the Day

We've mentioned that exercising causes the release of endorphins – or *happy chemicals*. These hormones put you in a good mood that can last for the rest of the day. On top of that, when you associate good feelings with working out, it makes you more likely to stick with the habit, making it a consistent part of your life.

Starting the morning with exercise can help you to have a better day. Exercise can boost creativity, help fight depression, and improve the ability to problem-solve.

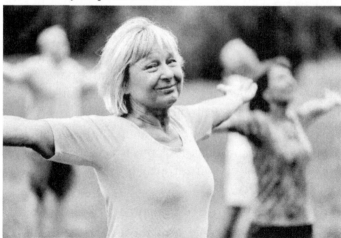

5. An older woman stretching in the morning.

4. It Increases Your Metabolism Rate

Working out first thing in the morning usually means you haven't gotten a chance to eat anything. In that case, there's hardly any sugar in your bloodstream for your cells to use for energy. Working out requires energy which is why we feel hungry after activity. Working out without eating means that the needed energy to perform the exercises will need to come from *somewhere*. Your muscle cells' response to this would be to break down and make use of *reserved fat* that is stored up in the body. This is a great way to aid in fat loss and can help target trouble areas where high accumulations of fat are stored.

Research has also shown that the resting metabolism rate is higher when you work out early in the morning than when you work out later in the day. This boost equates to your body burning more calories for energy during the day, and less will be available for your body to store as fat. Working out in the mornings while maintaining a calorie deficit would be a great place to start if you're trying to lose weight.

5. You Will Make Healthier Choices

Exercising in the morning gives you the feeling that you started the day down the right path. That can make it easier for you to refuse to do anything that spoils your progress. Since you started with being healthy, why not stick with it and make the whole day a positive success? The energy you get from working out puts you in a mood that makes you want to accomplish things and keep the positive momentum going. It could be easier for you to pass up on doughnuts or fries in favor of fruits or a salad to try and get the most out of your workout.

Exercising in the morning is like checking off the first thing on your daily health to-do list. It could be a subconscious effect but knowing that you've already started on the daily journey can help you ensure that every other aspect of your life supports your exercise habits. Bingo! The first step to a happier and healthier person.

6. It Can Help You Sleep Better at Night

Getting your heart rate and respiratory rate up by exercising in the morning can help you improve the quality of your sleep in the evenings. It could make it easier for you to wind down at night as you may be more tired after an energetic and productive day. You may go to bed earlier and experience a deeper, more restful sleep.

These benefits may help you decide that it's best to work out in the mornings. However, there are a few obstacles that may play more of a role depending on your lifestyle.

Working out in the morning usually entails waking up reasonably early, which is not conducive to everyone's sleep patterns or daily routine as you may be more of a late sleeper. If you wake up in the middle of your usual deep sleep, you may be reluctant to get up and even feel groggy for much of the morning.

Another critical factor in morning exercise is warming up. Warming up is essential to any workout, but it may be the most important in the morning. After sleeping all night with little movement, the body is often a little rigid first thing in the morning. So, to avoid injury, in this case, you would have to take more time to sufficiently warm up before getting to the workout. Going into primary training without a proper warm-up can strain your muscles before they're ready, causing injury and hindering all the benefits of an active lifestyle.

Therefore, while exercising in the morning is an excellent option with many advantages, it's important to recognize if it's feasible for you to get up and be active early. Remember to consider the extra time allotted for thorough morning warm-ups.

Benefits of Working Out in the Afternoons or Evenings

Given the benefits of working out in the mornings we discussed, you may be ready to set an earlier alarm for tomorrow or stick to your current morning routine. However, working out later in the day can set you up for an amazing tomorrow. Here are some reasons you might want to schedule a brisk walk or visit the gym in the afternoon or early evening.

1. It Can Help You Increase the Strength of Your Muscles

Depending on what kind of workouts you engage in and your exercise goals, afternoons and evenings may be better times for you. According to studies, peak muscle performance occurs in the afternoon and early evening due to fluctuating hormone levels and core body temperature. The same hormones that control feelings of tiredness at night and energy in the morning play a role in muscle strength. Based on when most people sleep, the body releases top levels of testosterone in the later afternoon and early evening.

Testosterone is the hormone responsible for strength in both males and females. This boost in the late afternoon would lead to greater strength and a better ability to lift more weight with less perceived effort during this time, for example. This feeling or period of increased capacity may also make it easier for some to perform exercises, especially if you're often groggy in the mornings.

Therefore, if your goal is to get stronger and harness maximum muscular strength, you may want to plan exercises for the latter part of the day.

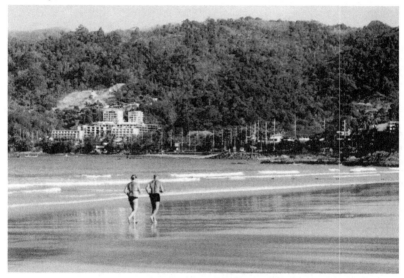

6. Older couple running at the beach.
https://pixabay.com/photos/beach-running-old-couple-people-2090181/

2. There Are Lower Chances of Injury

This point further bolsters one of the cons of working out in the mornings.

Your body temperature increases as the day progress and peaks in the afternoons. Higher temperature means better blood circulation, making it easier for you to perform the movements in your routines properly.

The fact that you've been moving all day translates to more flexible joints and muscles so that you can ease into your main workout faster. The day's movements and tasks serve as a natural warm-up that can help the body be more inclined to perform the exercises. This doesn't eliminate the need for a warm-up - but it could mean that you wouldn't have to spend a long time preparing your body before focusing on the main thing.

Afternoon workouts also receive the benefit of faster reaction time. In the late afternoon, blood circulation is better, and you are likely far from the fog and grogginess of the morning. This increase can be helpful in any exercise, especially when doing higher-intensity workouts or routines requiring switching quickly between different movements. You'll enjoy more fluid motions and be in better form, which will help you reap more rewards from your efforts.

These factors significantly reduce the chances of getting injured by overstretching your muscles or making a mental error when reacting during the workout.

3. You will have More Energy

Research has shown that we can last a bit longer when we exercise later in the day, even when we do so at a higher intensity. You may have more energy to do cardio and strength training in the afternoons or evenings rather than first thing in the morning. It makes sense because many people feel stiff - and even sluggish - during the morning.

Many people may also feel this way because they feel more energized later in the day after they've eaten and had coffee or tea. Getting this added boost from calories or caffeine may be the thing that does it for afternoon workout devotees.

The body needs time to wake up fully, and it could take up to an hour before you feel ready to exercise in the morning. Exercising in such a state could make you get tired faster because you may be making yourself do the movements with a body that's just not feeling up to it yet. It makes sense that you get tired faster than if you were working out once your body has already been "opened" up by other activities that you engaged in during the day.

4. You May be Able to Focus Better

Most people work out in the mornings; hence the gym is usually more populated then. A gym full of people can be energizing or motivating, but it also means waiting to use equipment and occasionally chatting with colleagues. For walkers, there may be more sidewalk and road traffic in the morning from those headed out to work and school. Because most people would be at work or school by then, hitting the gym later in the day allows you to avoid the crowds and focus on precisely what you're doing (with fewer distractions and delays).

It's important, especially when first starting out or trying to build a routine, to ensure these distractions are limited. Even a small streak of a week or two of focused exercise can be a powerful aid in creating a habit.

These days, many fitness centers are open 24 hours a day, allowing you to work out at a time that's most convenient for you. The goal is to ensure you get those workouts in and start feeling better.

5. It Can Really Help You Sleep Better

Your sleep shouldn't be affected if you time your workouts 3 to 4 hours before bedtime. It's true that performing exercise too close to bedtime is likely to energize you and may make it difficult to wind down and get good sleep. However, if you exercise a little earlier, by the time the endorphins and enhanced blood flow from the exercise return to normal, you could be surprised to find that it helps you sleep deeper and longer.

If you have some brain work to do in the evenings, the hours after a workout could be a great time to get them done, and you'll be amazed at how sharp your mind will be. However, when you're ready to go to bed, you'll fall asleep faster.

6. Less Stressed

The pressure of a long day might make you want to throw on some comfy clothes and flop on the couch – which is understandable – but evening exercise is a perfect way to de-stress. As mentioned earlier, working out releases a host of feel-good brain chemicals known as endorphins, lowering your stress levels and improving your mood.

Stress can seep in by the early evening, whether from work or the house being more crowded and hectic later in the day. Getting some exercise right around this time may release that tension or give you a healthy and productive break from the cause of the stress.

Another perk of working out later is the chance to use exercise to replace other unhealthy habits. Before dinner snacking, watching too much TV, or having an evening cocktail hour are replaceable habits that could be hurting your health goals. Try subbing these out with a happy-boosting workout and enjoy the doubled benefits.

As we mentioned in the previous point, you could take advantage of your brain's alertness after exercise to do some work or even play games that enhance your cognitive abilities even more, such as chess. This period of feeling better post-workout could become the best part of the day. You may find that you don't need some of those bad habits that were sabotaging your health.

7. The Next Day Will Be Amazing

One of the top benefits of an evening workout is that it sets you up for an amazing tomorrow. By getting rid of your daily stress and achieving better nightly sleep, you'll wake up feeling refreshed and ready to start a new day.

Although working out in the afternoons or evenings has many benefits, you may not be ready to ditch your morning routine. No worries! Keep this later workout option in mind for those days when you sleep in or have an early morning commitment and can't make it to the gym. For those curious or willing to try something different, give an afternoon exercise a try to see how it works for you.

Now that you know the difference between working out in the morning, afternoon, and night it's time to move on to other details like nutrition. Next, we'll review how to prepare and fuel your body and when to eat for workouts.

In conclusion, having considered the pros and cons of working out at various times, the important thing is *that you work out.* If you're always free around a particular time of the day, pick that time for your exercises; as much as possible, stay consistent. Also, remember that exercising too close to bedtime could adversely affect your sleep.

Working Out Fasted Versus Fed

Definitions: As the name implies, *working out fasted* is working out when you haven't had anything to eat in over four hours. *Working out fed* is when you're working out less than four hours after eating.

There are debates about whether it is safe to work out fasted – or if there are any additional benefits that come with working out fasted. Working out fasted can be a challenge for some as it will require the body to work harder as there won't be any easily accessible energy from food. The lack of food could cause some to feel dizzy or just plain zapped when attempting a fasted workout.

Disclaimer: working out more than six hours after your last meal is not for everyone. Your blood sugar is not only low at that time, but your body may also be in a ketosis state. Pre-existing health conditions may require some seniors to eat frequently and ensure their blood sugar does not drop too low, as in the case of fasting.

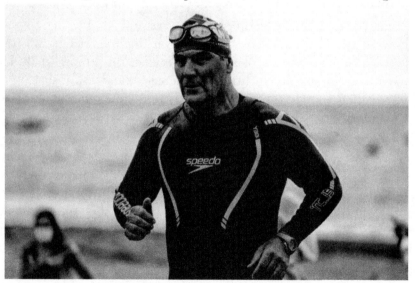

7. An older man running on the beach.
https://pixabay.com/photos/man-run-swim-older-athletes-7011342/

Ketosis is the state in which your body uses glycogen stores for energy; this could be detrimental to seniors as it would be a significant lack of carbohydrates. This lack would be a possible cause of low energy, especially for those who exercise or are just beginning a new routine.

The main benefit of working out fasted is that your body *burns fat faster*. Since there's no sugar in the bloodstream, your body calls upon fat reserves to use as a source of energy. Even this fat targeting may not necessarily translate to weight loss unless you maintain a calorie deficit. To lose weight and burn fat, you would have to consume fewer calories than you burn to reap the benefits of working out fasted. This would be if you're goal is to lose weight and reduce body fat and if you're participating in fasting or a keto diet.

Exercising in a fasted state is your decision, but the most important thing is that you listen to your body. If you feel faint or otherwise unwell, take a break – you may have overdone it. Keto diets and fasting are great tools for many to adjust their health, but they may be too advanced to start at the same time as a new workout routine. The primary goal should be getting the exercise in, especially when first starting.

What to Eat or Drink During and After a Workout

For some younger people, exercising and staying active isn't always easy. The same goes for those in their golden years, but exercise may have more of a positive impact on seniors' daily life enjoyment. Older adults who don't exercise could risk losing up to 80% of their muscle mass! That loss is not something we want, as losing muscle mass also means losing your independence.

However, something that may cause you to reconsider working out may be your energy levels. Energy levels may not always be what you wish as an older adult, and exercising without replenishing that energy does more harm than good. Improper nutrition before, during, and after workouts can lead to fatigue, sore muscles, and injury. So, the big question is, "what do you eat and drink to keep your energy up and repair muscle tissue?"

Drinks For Before a Workout

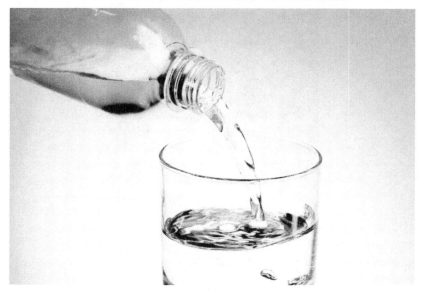

8. A glass of water being poured.

    1. Water: Water is the answer to most questions, and it's a great idea to go into a workout well hydrated. Drink some water leading up to and right before a workout to help improve hydration, stale cool and even improve endurance. Water costs no calories, and it really can only help the body. The only downside would be drinking too much and feeling full as you try to complete exercise movements.

    2. Electrolytes: Electrolytes are the powerful ingredient behind Gatorade and many squirt-style or powdered drink add-ins. Electrolytes are the nutrients we lose during exercise through sweat. Electrolytes can help ensure the nerve impulses travel properly throughout the body, such as using a muscle to move a weight. There have been many advances in electrolyte options, so be careful to choose the one suited to you. Some are high in carbohydrates which can provide energy but break a fast, while others have none.

    3. Coffee or Tea: Coffee and tea contain caffeine that can help power you through a workout. Caffeine can improve exercise capacity, make exercising more manageable, and improve recovery after exercise. When choosing a coffee or tea, remember that adding sugar or cream adds calories that can be beneficial for energy but may not aid in weight loss efforts.

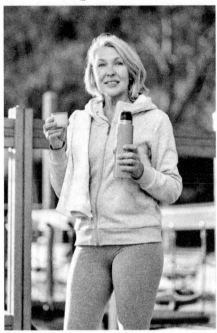

9. An older woman drinking coffee before her workout

4. Energy supplements: The purpose of an energy drink, pre-workout, or even an espresso before a workout would be to boost exercise capacity. The caffeine and other stimulants in energy drinks and pre-workouts push you through the workout. While these options can have a positive impact on workouts, it's best to consult a physician before attempting to use them.

Drinks During Workouts

1. Water: Once again, water is the hero of the workout. Sipping water during a workout can help keep you cool and give you a moment's rest to focus and catch your breath. It's important to stay hydrated, and a nice cool drink of water can help cool you off while exercising.

2. Electrolytes: Yes, electrolytes work here too. Essentially drinking an electrolyte beverage like Gatorade during the workout helps replace the nutrients your body is sweating out from exercising. The liquid will help to keep you hydrated and cool as you perform your movements.

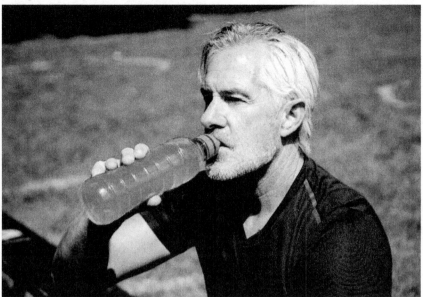

10. An older adult drinking an electrolyte beverage during exercise.

Drinks For After Working Out

1. Water: Of course, good old water tops the list! It's essential to stay hydrated while working out; drinking water is the easiest and cheapest way to hydrate your body. Staying hydrated can help keep joints loose and pain-free as well, leading to a stronger likelihood of continuing to exercise. Water serves other benefits, too, such as suppression of appetite, speeding up metabolism, and refreshing you during your workout.

2. Black and Green Teas: Both black and green teas contain antioxidants, and they can help increase the rate of muscle recovery and relieve muscle soreness after exercise. Green tea also helps increase metabolism and can be effective for weight loss. Tea is a hydrating and low-calorie drink option with the added benefits of antioxidants and caffeine.

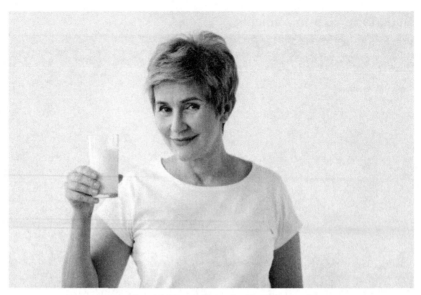
11. A senior drinking a glass of milk after exercising.

3. Low-fat Milk: Milk is a great source of protein and calcium. If you're not lactose intolerant, you can drink some milk after your workout to help repair the muscle tissues, boost energy, and aid in weight loss. Milk contains the building blocks the body needs to rebuild muscle and keep joints healthy. Milk also helps replenish the nutrients lost during a workout, such as sodium and potassium. **HINT**: Low-fat chocolate milk is also a tremendous balanced after-workout option and delicious too!

4. Non-dairy milk, such as almond, hemp, and oat milk, can also contain some protein, digestible fibers, and vitamins. Look for options that include these before selecting one at the store. These can serve to hydrate by replenishing fluids, replacing nutrients, and fortifying joints.

5. Protein Shake: It's necessary to get protein after a workout. Sometimes the quickest and easiest way is by drinking a protein shake. These can be made at home using a powder mixed with water or milk or bought premade. Ensure is an example of a premade protein shake that can serve as a perfect nutrient-dense snack after working out.

6. Beetroot Juice: Beetroots contain some natural chemicals called nitrates, and the body converts these nitrates to nitric oxide. There's some evidence to show that nitric oxide can help boost your performance during a workout, reduce muscle soreness after workouts, and help to lower blood pressure. Many stores sell beetroot that already has added juices to improve the flavor. Though beetroot juice can improve endurance during an exercise and may reduce soreness the next day, it is not a necessary part of exercise nutrition.

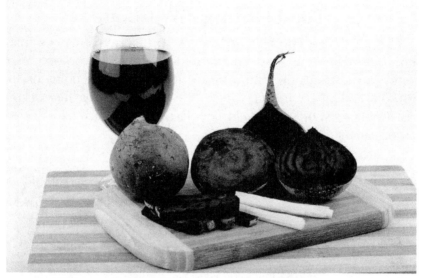

12. Beetroots and a glass of beetroot juice.
https://pixabay.com/photos/beetroot-vegetables-3434195/

There's no specific rule about what you must drink before, during, or after your workout. These options can help improve the results, but not all of them need to be used or are suitable for everyone. The most important takeaway is to stay hydrated regardless of whether you are working out or not.

Food Before Workouts

Meals: Eating before a workout needs to be tested by the individual. Eating and then waiting thirty minutes may provide you a good amount of sustained energy, but make you feel too sluggish to work out. Eating breakfast or lunch too close to a workout can also make you feel full and uncomfortable while trying to perform many movements.

Carbohydrates: Having a small snack of fast-digesting carbs such as a piece of white bread, banana, or crisp rice cereal can provide a powerful source of healthy energy. This energy will provide fuel for your muscles to perform and help them grow as well. It is recommended to use trial and error to ensure you like the fullness of eating a snack before working out.

Food During a Workout

Carbohydrates: Having a carb snack such as a crispy rice square during exercise can boost energy mid-workout. A workout snack could be a strong motivator to get to the halfway point of the workout and, afterward, may make the second half of the workout easier. The best options would be a fast-digesting carb like a cereal bar or banana.

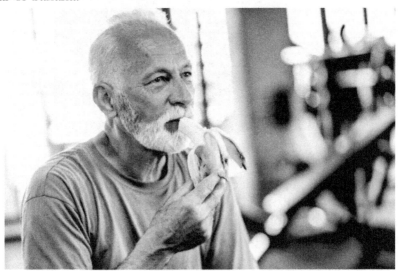

13. An older man eating a banana during his workout

Food After the Workout

It's advisable to eat soon after your workout - within an hour, which helps ensure you begin to regain your energy immediately. It is also prime time for your muscle tissues to start to absorb proteins and carbohydrates to repair themselves.

Meals: What you eat after a workout should ideally contain carbs, proteins, and a little fat because all these macronutrients are essential for your body's recovery process. There are some foods that are particularly good to eat as part of a meal after exercising, including sweet potatoes, grains, fruits, beef, pasta, chicken, eggs, nuts, or Greek yogurt.

Whether you're working out before breakfast, lunch, or dinner, food is always going to come up sometimes after working out, as the body will require calories. It's probably wise to try and plan a meal shortly after working out to help prevent overeating. Once your body has had some time to cool down, enjoy a nice high-protein meal.

Protein: Regardless of the timing of your workout, it's essential to have protein. Protein after the workout helps to rebuild the muscles and supports joint health. Protein shakes, protein bars, or just a few slices of lunch meat can serve as a filling and functional protein snack post-workout. Choose the option that works best for you and doesn't put a damper on your mealtimes.

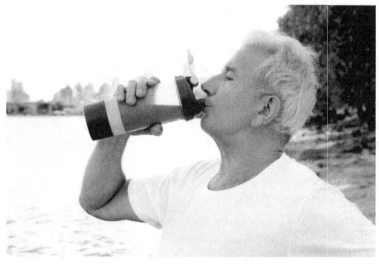

14. A senior drinking a protein shake.

You need to replenish energy and protein in your body after a workout in order to enjoy the benefits of that activity. Carbohydrates, proteins, and fats are all essential, though the specific amounts you need may vary with the kind of exercises you do. Listen to your body and if you feel hungry before or after a workout, have something to eat. And . . . don't forget to stay hydrated!

Chapter 3 How to Warm Up

It is a good thing that you have finally decided to take your health and fitness a little more seriously; congratulations on a healthy future! However, it is imperative to note that these routines shouldn't be taken lightly. Of course, there are easy exercises among them, but the fact is that they will all eventually be taxing on you, both physically and mentally. It will make life much easier if you start each routine, every day, by first warming up.

Children appear unharmed by sudden changes from sitting immobile to full-speed running. Clearly, that ability deteriorates as we age, so young and middle-aged adults – especially seniors – must warm up before engaging in rigorous activity or participating in sports. Adults seem to be more rigid, and joints certainly aren't as forgiving when we're older.

Warming up is an essential part of any exercise commitment. It is vital in several ways – even more so as you advance in age. It physically and mentally prepares you to begin any routine and helps you perform at your peak and finish a session strongly. An entire workout session could be wasted without first warming up as your body might not retain any gains. A session could also be swiftly ended by a sprain or strain if the body doesn't properly warm up before undertaking the exercise.

Stretching for flexibility in all your body parts is part of an ideal warm-up, but it takes more than stretching to warm up effectively; you must also engage your hearts and lungs to aid in readying your muscles and body. Two of the finest warm-ups you can engage in are taking a **short walk and marching in line** with exaggerated arm swings. If you cannot stand, a modification would be to sit up as straight as possible in a chair and perform the marching with your arms and legs. The movement will still wake the body up and promote positive circulation while seated.

To get in the workout mood, keep doing this for at least 10-15 minutes.

Let's look at some of the most effective warm-up exercises you can do as an older person. There are various types of warm-up exercises, such as seated exercises and sport-specific routines. There is at least one routine from each section, so experiment and find which type works best for you.

Shoulder Rolls

- (Useful Before Training: Back, Chest, Shoulders, Core, Push, Pull)

Benefits

How often do you stroke your neck in the hopes of getting a massage? Several times a day, if you're like most people. Shoulder rolls can relieve discomfort and stress in your neck by allowing nutrient- and oxygen-rich blood to flow to those tight neck muscles.

Shoulder rolls should be included in any stretching practice for those who frequently battle stiff shoulders and back muscles. Shoulder rolls require you to place your body in posture-correct positions, which can help you improve your posture.

Because sedentary employment contributes to bad posture and associated aches and pains, shoulder rolls are an excellent stretching exercise for people who work desk jobs.

Steps

1. Stand or sit tall with an open chest, neutral spine, and engaged core. Your shoulders should be kept back and down. Maintain a forward-looking position.

2. To begin, shrug your shoulders as high as you can toward your ears. Do not hunch your back, protrude your neck, or allow your shoulders to slump forward.

3. Squeeze your shoulder blades together and draw your shoulders back once you've shrugged as high as you can.

4. Pull your shoulders down by activating your mid-back.

5. Once you've reached the neutral starting posture, round your upper back slightly to press your shoulders forward while retaining a strong core.

6. Start a new shoulder roll by shrugging up again.

7. Perform 10 to 15 shoulder rolls, resting 30 seconds between sets. Three to five sets are a good goal.

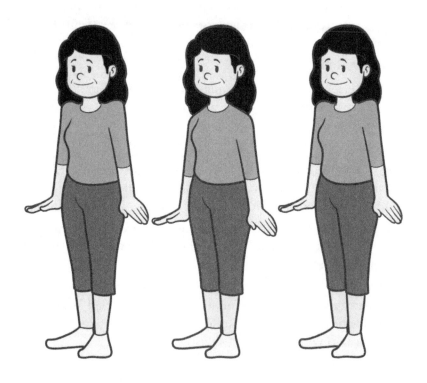

15. An older adult performing shoulder roll exercise

Shoulders Squeezes

- (Useful Before Training: Back, Chest, Biceps, Triceps, Shoulders, Core, Deadlifts)

Benefits

Ever lift a box off the table and feel a strain in the back middle or center of your back? This warm-up is good for activating the muscles of the mid-back and improving upper body movement mobility.

Use this before any upper body movements or before a task that involves reaching overhead or pulling. Shoulder squeezes will help open the chest while warming up the back. This could help improve stability when carrying something such as a box across a room.

Steps

1. Keep your arms by your sides and stand straight.

2. Alternately, bend your elbows 90 degrees and straighten your forearms in front of you.

3. Squeeze your shoulder blades together while pulling your elbows and arms back.

4. Squeeze symmetrically, making sure one shoulder blade does not come in faster or farther than the other.

5. Perform two sets of 10-20 reps.

These can be done seated, just like shoulder rolls.

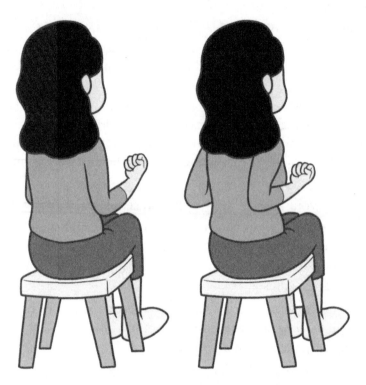

16. An elderly man performing Shoulder Squeeze

Neck Stretches

- (Useful Before Training: Back, Shoulders, Push, Pull)

Benefits

Neck stretches are like shoulder rolls in that they are very therapeutic. Neck stretches help to relieve tension in the neck and the muscles that support it.

By putting your neck through its full range of motion, you're preparing it to perform those movements again smoothly later.

These stretches should be used before any upper body movements. Surprisingly this is a good stretch to use before driving a car as it helps to warm the neck up in the case that you need to turn your head.

Steps

1. Keep your arms by your sides while standing straight.

2. Bend your neck back as far as you feel comfortable. Looking up at the ceiling is ideal.

3. Lean forward until your eyes are on your feet. Tuck your chin into your chest as much as you can.

4. Do this a total of 10-15 times.

5. Bend your neck and look to the left, then to the right, with your torso remaining straight ahead.

6. Do this a few times more.

7. Make around ten circles in each direction with your head.

   With the torso stationary, all your movements should be slow and controlled. You may perform these in a chair as well.

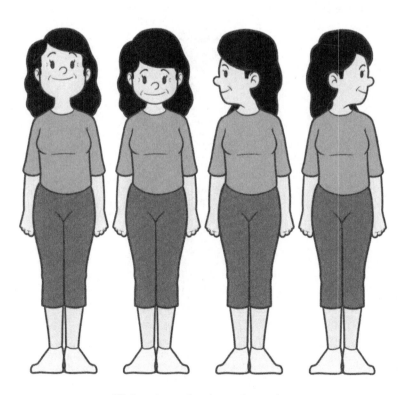

17. A senior performing neck stretches

Arm Swings

- (Useful Before Training: Back, Shoulders, Biceps, Triceps, Core, Chest, Push, Pull)

Benefits

Arm swings will help to open the chest, shoulders, and back. This movement will also help get the blood flowing through your arms and will likely increase your heart rate. This movement should be used as a warm-up for any pulling, pushing, or upper-body-focused exercise.

Steps

1. Stand tall with feet planted and arms straight by your sides.
2. Reach both arms back behind you until you feel a slight stretch.
3. Bring your straightened arms forward out in front of you to at least chest height if possible.
4. Repeat 15 times.

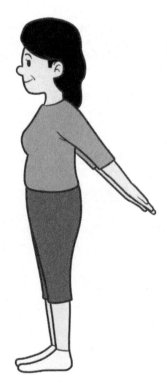

18. An elderly woman performing back-to-front arm swings.

Lateral Arm Swings

- (Useful Before Training: Back, Shoulders, Biceps, Triceps, Chest, Core)

Benefits

These should be used along with regular arm swings to increase circulation and warm up the upper body. This will help with motions that require you to raise your arms, reach across the body, or use your shoulder muscles.

Steps:

1. Stand tall and straighten your arms out to your sides with palms facing behind you.
2. Swing your straightened arms up and across each other, creating an "X" shape at chest level.
3. Return your arms to the original position by swinging them back down and behind your sides with palms facing the rear.
4. Repeat 15 times.

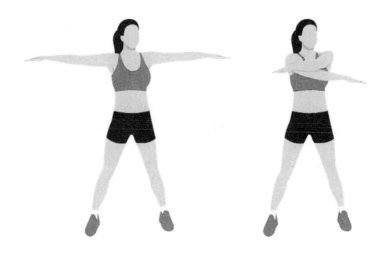

19. A woman performs lateral arm swings.

Wrist Circles

- (Useful Before Training: Biceps, Triceps, Chest, Shoulders, Back, Push, Pull)

Benefits:

You spend a lot of time typing on a computer, texting on your phone, or simply just writing with a pen. This repetitive motion can often lead to awkward wrist placement that can cause discomfort or tightness in the wrists. You may even sleep in a way that keeps the wrist from moving very much or holds it in an awkward position overnight.

These will be useful for anyone performing workouts using their arms or attempting to grip something. These can help prevent wrist injuries while performing daily tasks as well.

Steps:

1. Stand tall and hold your arms outstretched in front of you. Maintain balance. Modification: If arms can't be held outstretched, elbows can be kept at the sides and bent ninety degrees so that hands are kept straight in front of you. Perform the following steps from this position.
2. Without moving your arms, make outward circles with your wrists as if unwinding a spool of thread. Then repeat the motion making inward circles with your wrist as if winding a thread around a spool.
3. Perform eight outward circles and eight inward circles.

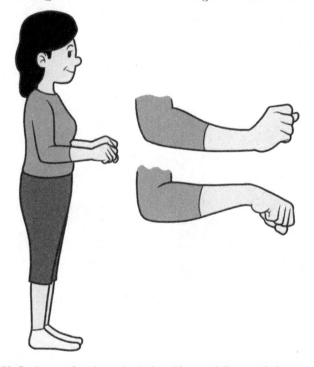

20. Seniors performing wrist circles with arms fully extended.

Leg Swings

- (Useful Before Training: Squats, Leg Extension, Leg Curls, Calf Raises, Deadlifts, Cardio)

Leg swings are a warm-up exercise to target the hips. Using a chair or wall for support, you'll loosen up your hips, active the glutes, and stretch the muscles of the front and back of the thigh.

These should be used before a walk, run, or lower body movements. They can also be used to loosen up the hips to aid in bending over with less tightness.

Steps:

1. Use your left hand to maintain equilibrium. Put your palm against a wall or grab the back of a table or chair.
2. Balance on the left leg and let the right leg hang loose
3. Swing your right leg forward and kick as high as possible without losing your balance or moving your left side.
4. After that, swing the leg back behind you. You won't be able to go back as far as you would like. Let the leg swing forward and backward comfortably without straining or forcing the motion.
5. Repeat this with the left leg.
6. Swing back and forth 10 times on each leg

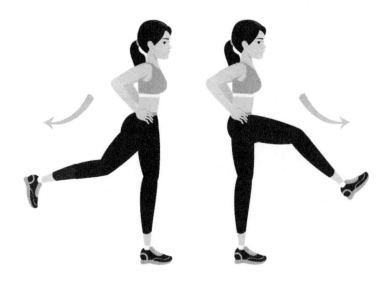

21. A woman performs back-to-front leg swings.

Lateral Leg Swings

- (Useful Before Training: Squats, Leg Extension, Leg Curls, Calf Raises, Deadlifts, Cardio)

Benefits:

Lateral leg swings are all about activating the lower body. They put the hips through a full side-to-side range of motion, which can help improve balance and relieve hip tightness.

Use lateral leg swings to warm up the hips, glutes, and legs before a walk or performing lower body exercises. This warm-up can also help improve stability and maintain mobility when moving or shifting from side to side.

Steps:

These are like leg swings in that they continue to activate and loosen the hips and legs.

1. Brace yourself with one arm extended against a wall or standing holding a chair in front of you for support.
2. Stand tall with the left leg and let the right leg hang free.
3. Keeping the leg straight, swing the right leg across the body until it crosses over the left foot.
4. Swing the straight right leg from the crossed position out to the right as far as you comfortably can.
5. Repeat this motion going from left to right.
6. Complete this movement 10 times before switching to the other leg.

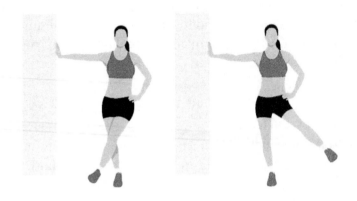

22. A woman performing a lateral leg swing.

Ankle Circles from a Sitting Position

- (Useful Before Training: Squats, Leg Press, Calf Raises, Deadlifts, Cardio)

Benefits:

Ankle circles will help warm up your legs and feet. This warm-up can help prevent injury from rolling the ankle or tripping from the feet and ankles not being fully activated.

This is a good movement to use before a walk, lower body exercises, or even before getting out of bed first thing in the morning. Ankle circles can also help relieve tension in the shin. Shin splints (that cause pain in the shin) can occur from long periods of standing or repetitive movements that eventually aggravate the tendons and muscles.

Steps:

1. Take a deep breath and sit up straight.
2. Cross your right leg over your left leg or extend your right leg. It's fine to extend your leg straight out or bend your knee so that your foot is just off the ground when you extend. These two positions will have different sensations.
3. Rotate your ankles in a circular motion counterclockwise, maintaining as much stability as possible throughout the rest of your leg. These may feel jerky; as best you can, smooth them out. Then repeat the circles again in the other direction.
4. Repeat the process ten times more in the opposite direction.

For an added challenge, raise and rotate both ankles simultaneously.

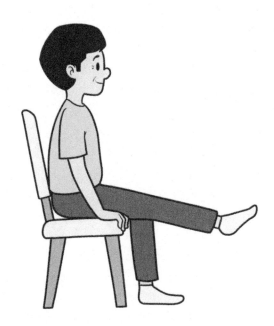

23. A man performing ankle circles in a sitting position.

Seated Hamstring Stretch

- (Useful Before Training: Squats, Leg Extension, Leg Curls, Calf Raises, Deadlifts, Cardio)

Benefits:

Your hips and knees are supported by strong, flexible hamstrings (on the back of the thigh), which help to prevent falls. They are a major source of power and are necessary for movement such as walking. Hamstrings can often become tight from lack of use, such as sitting or lying in the same position for long periods.

This exercise will loosen up tight hamstrings for more comfort and fluidity when walking. Perform this warm-up before lower body workouts or first thing in the morning upon sitting up in bed.

Steps:

1. Sit up straight in your chair or on the edge of the bed, feet flat on the floor and shoulder-width apart.
2. Extend your right leg, set your heel on the floor, and straighten your knee. (Your hands should be resting on your thighs.)
3. Slide your hands down your leg until a stretch is felt.
4. From the hips up, keep your back straight.
5. Allow your knee to bend slightly if it is stressed.
6. Maintain a 20-second hold. Deepening the stretch during the 20-second count is permissible but not required.
7. Switch sides and repeat.

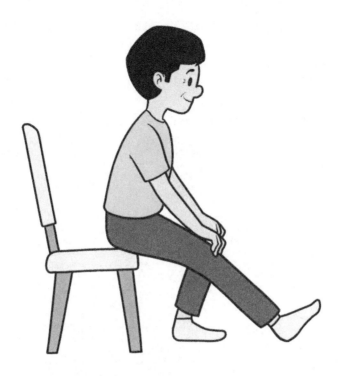

24. A man performing a seated hamstring stretch exercise

Knee Bends

- (Useful Before Training: Squats, Leg Extension, Leg Curls, Calf Raises, Deadlifts, Cardio, Leg Press)

Benefits:

The knees are often a source of discomfort for many as we use them so often. They are sensitive joints, and the cushion within the joint degrades over time.

The muscles of the legs are often tight from sitting or lying in one position at night or during the day. The knee bend helps to warm up the muscles with a light stretch while moving the knee in its natural direction when bent.

Knee bends can help prime the knee joint while warming up the muscles of the leg. This can help prevent tightness or strain when performing lower body exercises, going for a walk, or just getting up and down out of a chair.

Steps:

1. Stand tall and bend one knee while keeping the other straight. This will lift your foot up off the ground and put it slightly behind you.
2. Once a stretch is felt in the thigh, return the foot to a natural standing position.
3. Repeat the movement ten times for each leg.

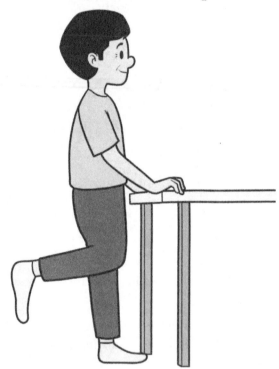

25. A older adult performing a knee bend.

Hip Lifts from a Sitting Position

- (Useful Before Training: Squats, Leg Extension, Leg Curls, Calf Raises, Deadlifts, Cardio)

Steps:

1. Sit in your chair with your back pressed firmly against the chair's back.
2. Grip the chair's sides with your hands.
3. Lift your right hip and knee, keeping them in place for 10 to 20 seconds.
4. Repeat three times on each side.

Slide forward in the chair to get a slightly different feel. Alternatively, cross your legs and elevate your hip and upper leg.

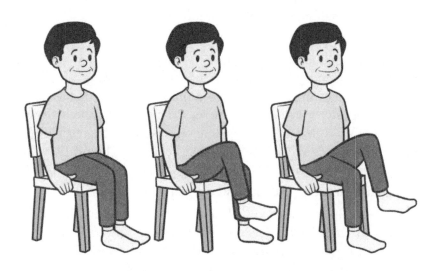

26. An older man performing seated hip lifts

The Benefits of Warming Up

1. Heart Benefits

The purpose of a warm-up is to get your cardiovascular system ready for a workout; your muscles will contract more fiercely and relax more quickly. This increase in heart rate improves the body's ability for strength and quickness. The heart also responds to warm-up movements by pumping more blood more quickly. Warming up your cardiovascular system makes it easier to meet the higher demands of a workout and prevents a blood pressure surge or feelings of unsteadiness from beginning too abruptly.

2. Increases the safety of the workout

Your brain and body must operate in unison for a workout to be successful and safe. Your nervous system needs to adjust to the change in activity and strain you'll be putting on the body during exercise. Warming up informs your body that it must prepare for a more strenuous activity than what it was doing previously, making your workouts safer and more efficient.

3. Helps to raise body temperature

When your body's temperature is slightly raised, it performs better. In the morning, warming up helps increase your body temperature, allowing you to notice a minor boost in performance. Getting the body "warm" means increased circulation and activation of muscles. Warming up before exercise aids in calorie burn as well. Getting into the "zone" with increased heart rate, blood flow, and maybe even working up a little sweat heats up and primes the body.

4. Increases muscle pliability and oxygen delivery

Warming up increases your blood flow and muscular flexibility. When your muscles have been through their range of motion or activated with a warm-up, they are less likely to be surprised. When a muscle is surprised by a movement in a workout, it could result in an injury such as a pulled muscle. Warming up improves your body's ability to provide oxygen and nutrients to functioning muscles, allowing them to perform better.

5. Improves cohesion

Your nervous system communicates with muscles more effectively when it is adequately prepared. Your body responds with quicker reaction times and swifter motions when the nerve-to-muscle pathways communicate clearly. Warming up before exercise can improve exercise performance and allow for more difficult sessions with less risk of injury.

6. Increases mental acuity

Stressed seniors are less likely to do well during their workouts. Stress causes them to become distracted and even slower. They also lose focus on the task at hand, become sloppy, and occasionally may be harmed. It's also a good idea to psychologically prepare for an exercise by clearing your thoughts, improving your attention, and evaluating your skills and approach; warming up before exercise provides mental preparation in addition to physical benefits.

7. It helps you exercise longer by increasing your endurance.

Your body's capacity to exercise is harmed when lactic acid builds up in your blood. Lactic acid can build up faster in the bloodstream without a warm-up, making working out nearly impossible in the first few minutes. On the other hand, warming up can aid your body's energy systems to adapt to the increasing demands and reduce lactic acid accumulation, allowing you to exercise longer and harder.

8. It fires up metabolism and energy production.

During a warm-up, your body produces more hormones that regulate energy levels. More carbs and fatty acids are accessible for energy use due to this hormonal balance. Thus, warming up before exercise helps increase metabolism and enhances energy.

9. Warm-up increases core activation and joint stability.

Warming up your joints, particularly the hips, knees, ankles, and shoulders, helps improve your range of motion. A senior's capacity to move efficiently is limited by aging or less mobile joints, reducing power and causing one to slow down. Injuries to stiff joints are also common. Warming up the glutes, spine, abdominals, hip flexors, and back muscles helps your body stay solid and balanced during the workout.

10. Assists with objections

On days when you don't feel like exercising, a warm-up might help you get started. Warm-ups can be a fantastic motivator! A senior should warm up for at least 10 minutes.

Note: a warm-up can also be used to put your body that has been injured or sick to the test. Warming up can prepare the body for the day and help prevent the chances of injury for seniors.

Try to perform these stretches even on days when a workout doesn't seem likely.

Dangers of Skipping Warm-Up

1. You may get injured.

You may have escaped damage today, but omitting a regular warm-up increases the possibility of getting a muscle strain or other injury. Take 10 minutes to warm up before working out; otherwise, you risk an injury that could set you back for weeks. The purpose of the warm-up is to prepare the body for movement and activity, which is the goal of continuing to exercise as a senior.

According to the Mayo Clinic, incorrect loading of the joints and muscles during a large lift is one of the most common causes of acute muscle strains. On the other hand, warming up before exercise prepares your body to load the proper muscles and follow movement patterns that help you avoid injury.

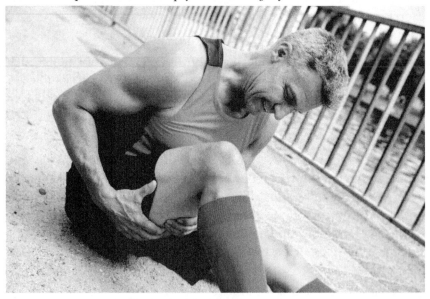

27. A senior injured during a workout.

For example, when warming up for deadlifts (which requires bending the hips and knees to reach down before lifting the weight up), you should first practice the hip hinge action with a move like the *good morning exercise* (standing tall with legs together and bending over at the hips only until the body forms close to a 90-degree angle*)*, which teaches you how to load your hips, buttocks, core, and back effectively.

2. Your Results May Be Affected

According to chiropractor R. Alexandra Duma (Team USA's sports chiropractor of New York City's recovery and wellness studio, FICS), warming up your muscles before a workout helps improve the body's core and muscular temperature. "Think of it like a warm-up for your car on a chilly winter day – it just performs better," Duma explains. Your joints become more flexible as the temperature of your muscles rises, increasing your range of motion.

But don't just do it for the sake of it; working hard during your warm-up may help you perform better during the big event, according to research. (In other words, you'll squat deeper and carry heavier weight)

Types

Active warm-ups

Active warm-ups are the most popular, and if they are not too strenuous, they have been found to boost performance. They involve moving the body through motions. Active stretching is when a muscle is contracted so that another is stretched. Done properly, they help the body use oxygen more efficiently while not draining its energy reserves and increasing flexibility. Experts frequently recommend that a sport-specific warm-up follow a basic aerobic warm-up.

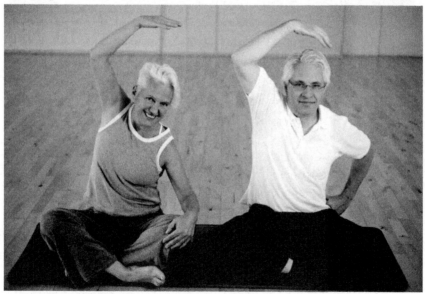

28. Seniors participating in an active warm-up stretch.

Passive warm-ups

Passive warm-ups involve increasing your body temperature through external sources like a hot bath or sauna to loosen the body up. This strategy achieves many of the same benefits as active warm-ups while avoiding tiredness. However, it does not deliver all the advantages of vigorous active warm-ups. You might try a passive warm-up in combination with some stretching.

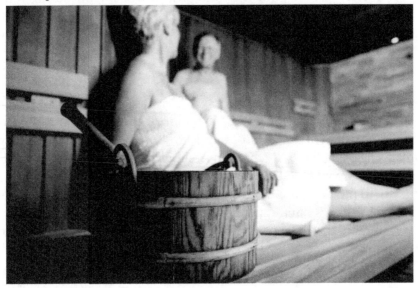

29. Seniors using the sauna as a passive warm-up

Static Stretches

Static stretching is a type of stretching that involves stretching on the spot with no rotational limb movement. Most warm-up regimens used include static stretching, which consists of holding a position for 30 to 90 seconds. Static warm-ups can be used to loosen up tight muscles through stretching, but this type of stretching is especially beneficial after exercising. *Ballistic stretching* or bouncing during a stretch should not be performed as it has lost favor with experts due to the risk of injury.

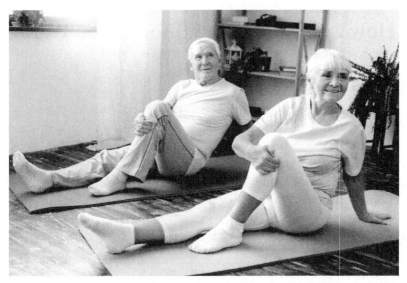

30. Seniors practicing static stretching

Dynamic stretching

Dynamic stretching includes moving the body to simulate the upcoming action. It preps the muscles and joints that will be used for a focused workout movement. Walking or lunges are common warm-up exercises for runners.

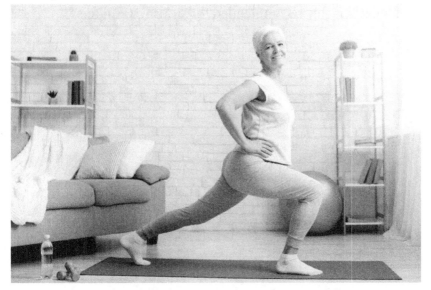

31. A senior lunging as part of a dynamic stretch warm-up

How Long and Often Should You Warm up?

Warm-up Techniques that Work

When it comes to warming up, how long should you spend? Professional athletes typically prepare for a game or competition for a long time. Tennis professionals, for example, practice for an hour before a match. Warming up muscles is not all professional athletes do; they're also practicing *a set of moves* (where they go through the motions of the movements they are about to perform for the sport).

Warm-ups for seniors should last at least 10-15 minutes and be performed right before exercise. Many warm-up exercises are beneficial to everyday activities and general health and, therefore, can be performed daily. Remember not to overdo your warm-up, and if you feel too tired, don't push yourself through further exercises.

Taking your time to engage in warm-up exercises before embarking on any of your choice workouts is a good practice with numerous benefits, especially for seniors. To aid in injury prevention and get your body and mind motivated and focused for exercise, it is highly recommended to perform warm-ups.

Chapter 4 Work Your Back and Biceps

There are a variety of advantages to incorporating a back and biceps workout. The reason these two muscle groups are focused on at the same time is that they are both used in many of the same exercises. For instance, pulling workouts that use and build your back muscles also use the biceps muscles as a supplementary source of strength.

Because the biceps are an auxiliary muscle group for many back workouts, you'll be strengthening your back and biceps simultaneously. Your training routine largely depends on your fitness goals. Conventional strength-exercising procedures advise exercising larger muscles first, then smaller muscles. This strategy is meant to make exercise easier and reduce the risk of injury. The larger muscles like the back will be able to endure more weight and will last longer than smaller muscles like the bicep. While this strategy is beneficial, evaluate your physical fitness goals and which muscle sets you would like to focus on while scheduling your exercise.

Integrating back and biceps into a single workout also enables older adults to perform the activity using popular workouts in one session, eliminating the need to divide them into specific sessions and giving them an extra rest day.

Back and biceps exercises involve pulling and lifting. These will be beneficial in everyday movements like opening doors, holding boxes or bags, or grabbing and moving things closer.

Some examples of workouts in this category are:

Dumbbell Curls: Which requires you to lift weight in front of your body using just your arms.

Lat Pulldown: involves getting into a seated position and reaching up to pull a bar on a cable with resistance from weights down to your chest.

Supermans: Involve lying face down on the floor and raising up your arms and legs.

Home Workout for Back and Biceps with No Equipment

These are workouts that you can easily do in your own home. They do not require gym equipment (unless you consider a mat or your yoga pants as "equipment"). You also do not need a friend, relative, or anyone around to accomplish them. They are simple and straightforward movements that can be completed by most individuals.

Supermans

Steps:

1. Lie face down on the floor with your face looking straight down at the ground.

2. Reach your arms palms down overhead as far as you can (like Superman flying).

3. Let legs lie naturally with the tops of feet facing the ground.

4. Inhale. Engage your back and shoulders, squeeze your glutes and lift your extended arms and legs up off the ground. Your chest and part of your thighs should come off the ground as well.

5. Hold your body in the raised position for 15 seconds if possible before lowering back down. Exhale.

6. Be sure to keep your head and neck straight by looking at the ground.

7. Rest for 30 seconds before repeating the movement for 3 repetitions

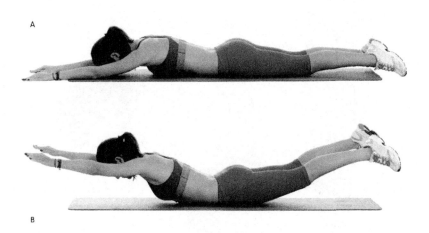

32. A woman performing Supermans

Good Mornings (Hip Hinge)

1. Stand with hands on hips with feet slightly wider than hips

2. Keep your neck neutral and hands and shoulders firm as you bend at the waist.

3. Inhale. Slowly bend over until your upper body is as close to parallel with the floor as you can achieve. Your glutes and hips should be thrust backward when you complete this movement.

4. Slowly exhale. Keep your back straight and engage your glutes, lower back, and hamstrings (back of the thigh muscle). Raise your upper body back to the starting position.

5. Repeat this movement for three sets of 10 repetitions. Rest 30-60 seconds between each set.

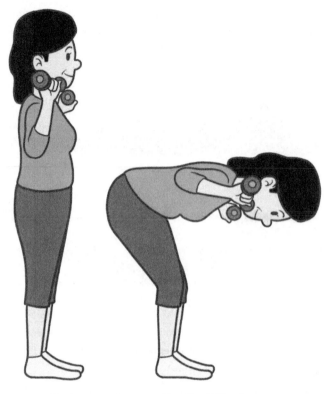

33. A woman demonstrating Good Mornings.

Standing Arm Lifts

1. Stand with feet slightly wider than hips and bent knees. Bend forward into a hip hinge position, so the hips are back, and the upper body is supported in a forward bend at about a 45-degree angle.

2. Keep your neck neutral with eyes looking at the floor directly in front of them. Pull your shoulders back and down and brace yourself with your stabilized core.

3. Hold your extended arms out in front of you. Exhale as you pull your arms back like bird wings until they form a "T" with your body. Inhale as you slowly lower your arms back down.

4. Exhale. Raise your arms up until they align with your body to form a "Y". Inhale. Slowly lower your arms back down.

5. Exhale. Raise your arms straight up until they are aligned with your body, and your biceps are by your ears to form an "I". Inhale. Slowly lower arms back down to in front of the body.

6. Repeat this series of three raises for three sets of 8 repetitions, with 60 seconds of rest between sets.

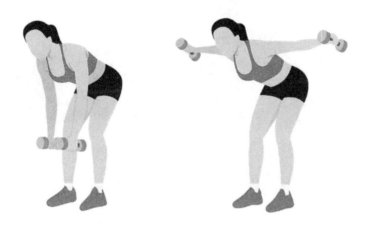

34. A woman performs a "T" Arm Lift with small dumbbells

Arm Raises (lying down)

1. Lie on your back with your legs bent and feet planted. Keep your arms down by your sides with palms on the ground.

2. Exhale. Slowly raise one arm at a time until it is extended straight out in front of you at about chest level. Inhale. Lower the arm back down to the floor.

3. Complete three sets of 10 repetitions for each arm. **Note:** You will feel this working your shoulders as well.

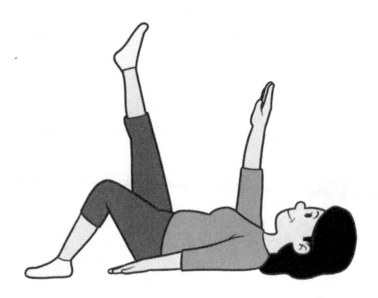

35. A woman performing a Lying Arm Raise

Biceps Isometric Hand Press

1. Stand up straight and place your hands together in front of you in a prayer position.

2. Turn prayer hands so fingertips are pointing directly away from the chest.

3. Bend elbows slightly to about a 45-degree angle, so arms aren't fully extended or too close to the body.

4. Exhale while pressing hands together without allowing any movement in the arms and hold for 10 seconds. Inhale.

5. Repeat hold for three sets with 30 seconds of rest between sets

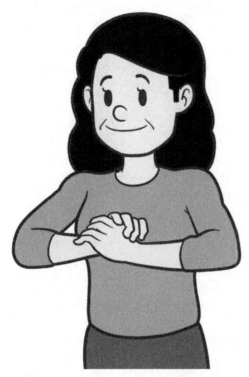

36. A woman performing an Isometric Biceps Hold.

No Weight Curl

1. Stand tall with shoulders back and arms down at your sides. Make two fists and hold your hands so your palms are facing in front of you.

2. Exhale. Slowly raise arms up to 90 degrees by contracting the bicep and bending at the elbow.

3. Hold your arms at the top for 5 seconds. Breathe out and slowly lower them down to fully extended at your sides.

4. Repeat this for three sets for 10 repetitions with 30-60 seconds rest between sets.

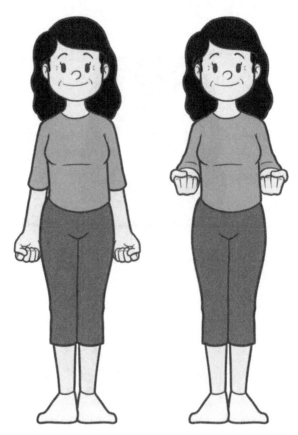

37. A woman performing Bicep Curls with no weights.

Home Workout for Back and Biceps with Equipment

These exercises can be done at home using purchased home gym equipment or things around the house as substitutes. Be sure to test out the weights or resistance bands before buying them to make sure they are a suitable weight for your current fitness level. You can always buy lighter ones and use them until you progress to something heavier.

If no gym-specific equipment is purchased, then other household items can often be used in place to achieve similar results. These will just have to be collected and tested for safety and practicality of use in an actual workout.

Bent-Over Row

Option: This exercise can also be completed with a barbell or household substitutes (like a loaded bag or laundry bin).

1. Grab a pair of dumbbells. These will probably be a little bit heavier than those used for arm exercises since they will be using your back, which is a larger muscle group, and your arms.

2. Stand with feet shoulder-width apart and bend over at the waist at about a 45-degree angle. The dumbbells will be in your hands, held down at arm's length with inward-facing palms.

3. Use your back while squeezing shoulder blades together to pull your bent elbow up and back behind your back. This will pull the dumbbells up and in – so they are resting on either side of your midsection. Pause for a second at the top before lowering the weights back down to the starting position.

4. Repeat this for three sets of 8-10 reps with 30-60 seconds of rest between sets.

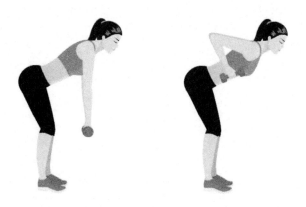

38. A woman demonstrating a Bent Dumbbell Row.

Deadlift

Option: This exercise can be done with s set of dumbbells, a barbell, or something with some weight that can be gripped from around the house, such as a loaded backpack or laundry basket.

1. Stand tall with chest up and feet shoulder-width apart. Shoulders should be pulled back, and there should be a slight arch in the back.

2. Dumbbells should begin in your hands in front of your thighs with palms facing towards the body.

3. Bend down by hinging at the hip and bending the knees. The back should be kept straight (don't let it round), and the neck should be in a neutral position with eyes looking in front of you.

4. Keeping arms straight, lower the dumbbells down right in front of your legs as you hinge your hips and bend your knees. If you can get to parallel, that's great, but otherwise, just lower until you feel the stretch in your lower back and hamstrings.

5. Pull the weights up by thrusting your hips forward to their natural position and pushing through your feet. You should stand in a straight-up position with the weights in front of your thighs.

6. Repeat for three sets of 8 reps with 60 seconds of rest between sets.

6. Start with a light weight and progress to heavier once a foundation of strength and balance has been built for this movement.

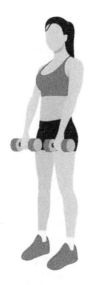
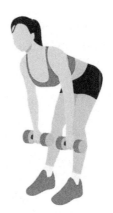

39. A woman performing a Dumbbell Deadlift.

Bent-Over Lateral Raise

Tip: Start light with a light weight or even begin this exercise with no weights as a warm-up. It is in an awkward position, and there may not be much strength built up when first beginning.

1. Sit on the edge of a sturdy chair or on the edge of an exercise bench. Keeping a 90-degree angle in the knees, plant your feet firmly on the ground. Grasp a light dumbbell in each hand and keep them hanging down on the outside of the thighs hanging down below them.

2. Bend over at the waist until the chest is close or touching the top of the thighs. Keep neck neutral. The inside of your forearms should be against the outside of your thighs, and the weights will be hanging down at about calf level.

3. Keep a slight bend in the elbow and focus on trying to bring your shoulder blades together in the middle of your back as you

exhale and lift the weights out and up and out to the sides. The weights should raise to above thigh height. If you cannot raise them this high, it's okay to raise them to a lesser degree that feels comfortable.

4. Pause briefly at the top of the movement before breathing in and slowly lowering the weights down to hang below the outside of your thighs.

5. repeat this for three sets of 8-10 repetitions. Rest 30-60 seconds between sets.

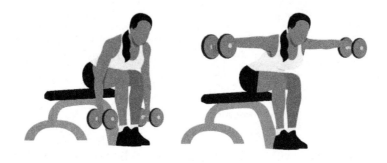

40. A woman demonstrates a Seated Bent-Over Lateral Raise.

Dumbbell Bicep Curl

1. Stand tall with shoulders back and arms down at your sides. Hold the dumbbells at your sides or slightly resting on the front of your thighs. Your palms should be facing in front of you with thumbs away from the body.

2. Slowly raise arms to 90 degrees by contracting the bicep and bending at the elbow.

3. Hold your arms at the top for a second before slowly lowering them down to fully extended at your sides or slightly resting on your thigh.

4. Repeat this for three sets for 8-10 repetitions with 30-60 seconds of rest between sets.

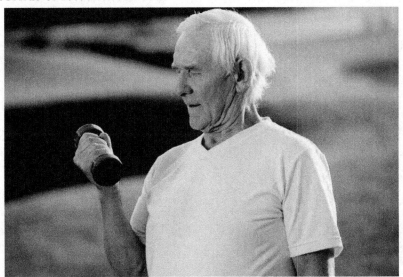

41. An older man performs dumbbell biceps curls.

Resistance Band Row

For this exercise, you will need a resistance band. This can be one with a handle or one without. These bands come in different weights and can be purchased from many big box stores or online. Purchasing a set with multiple weights can serve as a powerful tool for progressing while also providing the option to use the appropriate weight.

1. Attach a resistance band to an anchor either by looping it around, fastening it with a provided clip, or tying it on. This anchor point can be overhead, midbody, or on the floor.

2. Depending on the method the band was attached, this move will either use one arm at a time or both if two handles or ends are available.

3. Stand with shoulders back and legs shoulder-width apart, far enough for the band to almost be taut.

4. Contracting the mid-back muscles, pull the band towards you until your elbow is bent and either by your side or behind you. Hold for a second.

5. Slowly return to the starting position.

6. Repeat this movement for three sets of 10 reps. Rest 30-60 seconds between sets.

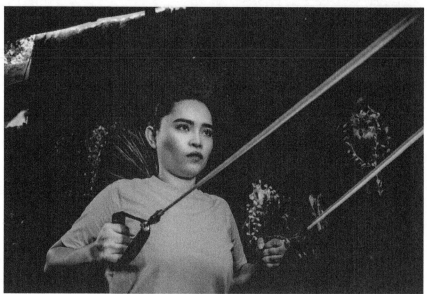

42. A woman performs a Resistance Cable Row.

Rope Pull

Option: This exercise can also be done from a sturdy chair. Sit upright and try to keep the spine straight when pulling from this position.

1. Tie or attach a sheet or rope to something heavy like a dumbbell, full laundry basket, or backpack.

2. Stand with feet slightly wider than hip-width apart as far away from the object as possible with the rope in your hands. Bend the knees and hinge the hips back slightly.

3. Pull the object towards your body using your back by reaching hand over hand on the rope and pulling the elbow back behind the body. Pulling the elbow back will help engage your *lats* or mid-back

muscles.

4. Return the weight to the starting position and repeat the pulling process. Do this for 4-6 sets with 30-60 seconds of rest between sets.

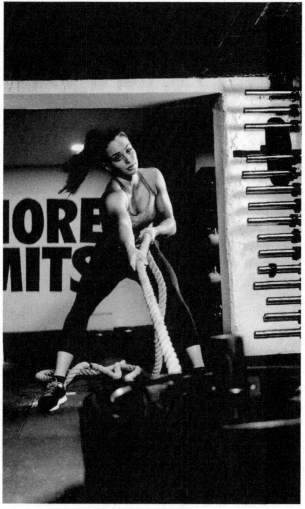

43. A woman performs a Weighted Rope Pull

Gym Workout for Back and Biceps

The gym is an excellent way to start and maintain an exercise routine. The gym offers a safe place with easy-to-use equipment ready to go. For these exercises, I will focus on gym machines that can make exercise easier and more convenient.

The machines at the gym usually have instructions written on them that explain how to perform the exercise properly. These can be very helpful, but if you cannot understand them, find a gym attendant and do not be afraid to ask for help.

Lat Pulldown

Option: There are other handles that can be attached to the pulldown machine and used instead for similar results. Similar machines also allow the pulldown motion with a different-looking setup but target the same muscles.

1. Adjust the pin in the weights to a suitable amount. Always start with a lower weight to warm up and for safety, and then increase it afterward if necessary.

2. Select the long bar attachment for the pulley system and carefully attach it.

3. Sit down in the seat and adjust the leg restraint so that it is tight on the top of the thighs. The shins should be against the leg pads below, and the feet should be planted on the floor.

4. Grab the bar while standing and carefully pull the weight down with you as you get secured into the seat restraint.

5. Adjust your grip on the bar so that your hands are slightly wider than shoulder length apart. Lean back very slightly and look ahead or slightly upwards towards the machine.

6. Open the chest up and keep the chin tucked slightly for safety. Lead with your elbows as you pull the bar down to the chin or lower if possible. Pull your elbows down and back behind the body to engage the back muscles. There should be a squeeze in the mid-back at the bottom of the pull movement.

7. Pause briefly at the bottom of the movement before slowly letting the bar return to the top. Allow the bar to return upwards until your arms are fully extended above you before pulling the weight down again.

8. Do this for three sets of 10 repetitions with 30-60 seconds of rest between sets.

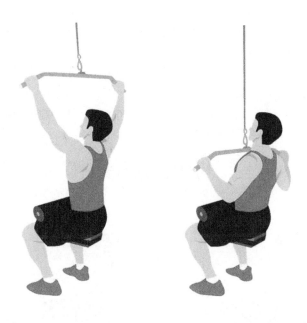

44. A man performs the seated lat pulldown.

Seated Cable Row

Option: There are multiple handles that can be attached to the cable row that will provide a workout for the back. The different handles will slightly alter the focus of the movement.

1. Adjust the weight using the pin system on the machine located near its center. Choose a weight that's right for you as it can always be increased later. Select the handle you'd like to use

2. Sit in the seat with feet planted on the supports in front and knees bent. Keep the spine in an upright position and keep the shoulders neutral. Bend the knees and lean slightly forward to grab the handle in front of you.

3. Extend your arms and grab the handle securely. Extend the knees and use your legs to position yourself back in the seat and in an upright position while holding the weight with the cable pulled tight in front of you.

4. Keep your chest up and your neck neutral as you look straight ahead. Pull the cable handle back towards your abdomen, leading with your elbows. Pinch the shoulder blades together to engage the back. The elbows should end up bent and slightly behind the body at the end of the movement.

5. Slowly let the cable retract until your arms are fully extended again.

6. Repeat this motion for three sets of 10 reps with 30- 60 seconds of rest between sets.

GYM WORKOUT
SEATED CABLE ROW

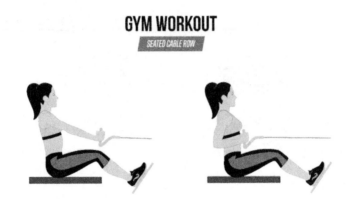

45. A woman demonstrates the Seated Cable Row.

Straight Arm Pulldown

1. For this exercise, you will need to find the cable machine that is meant to be stood in front of. Adjust the weight to a lighter weight to begin.

2. Attach a straight bar attachment to the cable machine and adjust the height so the cable is at the top. The bar will be hanging down in front of you as you stand facing the machine,

3. Stand with feet slightly apart and arms grasping the bar about shoulder-width apart. Arms will remain fully extended throughout the movement. Pull the bar down so the cable is taut and your arms are extended out slightly less than parallel to the ground.

4. Push hips back and lean the upper body slightly forward. Keep the back straight and neck neutral. Exhale. Pull

straightened arms down and pull the bar down and towards the top of the thighs. Keep the movement smooth and slow.

5. Pause for a second with the bar touching the top of the thighs. Breathe before slowly lowering the weight until your arms are almost parallel to the floor.

6. Repeat for three sets of 8-10 reps. Rest 30-60 seconds between sets.

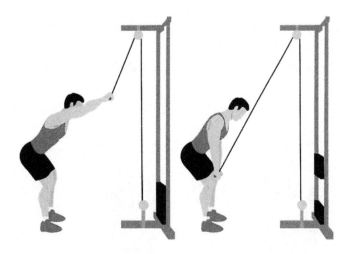

46. A man performs the Straight Arm Pulldown.

Cable Curl

Option: Various attachments can be used for the cable curl. These include the rope attachment, straight bar, or EZ curl bar (the squiggly or flying bird-shaped bar)

1. Find the same cable machine that you use for Straight Arm Pulldowns whose height can be adjusted.

2. Attach the EZ bar curl attachment to the cable pulley. Adjust the height so the cable connects to the bottom of the machine.

3. Stand with feet planted shoulder-width apart. Grasp the handle with palms up and thumbs away from the body. Pull the bar until arms are outstretched and the bar is resting against the top of the thigh area.

4. Maintain a straight back and keep the arms in line with the body. Exhale and bend only at the elbows, squeeze the bicep, and pull the cable up until the elbow is at least at a 90-degree angle. Hold the cable there for a second.

5. Inhale as you slowly lower the cable down to your thighs.

6. Repeat this movement for three sets of 10 reps. Rest 30-60 seconds between sets

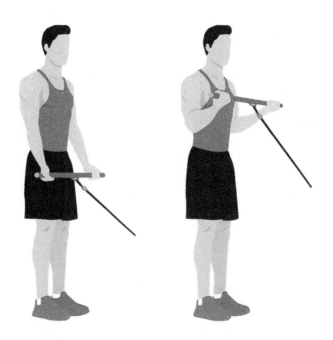

47. A man demonstrates the Cable Bicep Curl

Partner Workout for Back and Biceps

Supermans (Flying Together)

Note: Partners can take turns dictating when both raise and lower arms, or they can compete to see who can hold them up the longest before lowering.

1. Find an area of the floor where two partners can comfortably lay down and stretch out.

2. Both seniors lie face down with arms outstretched overhead and palms on the floor. The legs should be extended, and the tops of the feet should be facing the ground.

3. Partners should both exhale while contracting or squeezing the back, glutes, and shoulders, simultaneously lifting arms and legs up off the ground. Partners should both look like Superman flying with arms and legs outstretched.

4. Pause briefly at the top or until one of the partners says down. Inhale and slowly lower your arms and legs back down to the ground.

5. Repeat for two sets of 8-10 reps while varying hold durations at the top of the movement. Rest 30-60 seconds between sets.

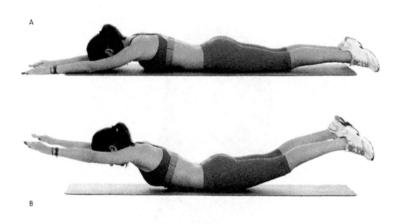

48. A woman performs Supermans

Partner Cable Row

For this exercise, you will need a resistance band, handled resistance cable, or two sets of handled resistance cables. The goal is for one senior to be the anchor while the other pulls or for seniors to take turns pulling as they provide resistance for each other.

This exercise can be completed sitting or standing for safety and based on the seniors' strength.

1. Grab a looped resistance band. If it is a larger loop, that would be preferred. Partners should each grab an end and face each other.

2. Step back until the band is taut between the partners. Stand with legs shoulder-width apart and grip the band with both hands. Make sure both partners are in a sturdy position.

3. Keeping a straight back. Exhale and think about pulling the elbows back and together towards the center of your back. Leading with the elbows, pull the cable towards your body. The elbows will bend as the cable is pulled, and the elbows should end somewhere close to behind the back.

4. Inhale and slowly let the band return to the starting position.

5. Repeat this move for three sets of 8-10 repetitions. Rest 30-60 seconds between sets.

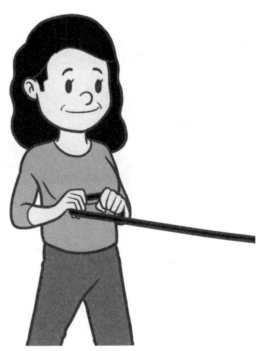

49. A woman and her partner demonstrate resistance cable rows.

Partner Band Curls

For this exercise, you'll need a resistance band, a handled resistance band, or a looped resistance band.

1. One partner will stand with the resistance band under the middle of their feet.

2. The other partner will grasp the other end of the band or the handles. Step back from the partner until the cable is close to taut.

3. Grasp the handles or band with palms facing up and thumbs away from the body at about waist height. Exhale while contracting the biceps and bending only at the elbows. Pull the handle up until the elbow is at least a 90-degree angle.

4. Pause briefly at the top of the curl before breathing in. Slowly lower the band back down so that hands are at about waist height.

5. Repeat for three sets of 10 reps. Rest 30-60 seconds between sets. Partners should either alternate sets or switch positions after three sets have been completed.

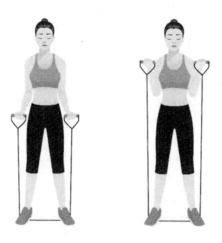

50. A woman demonstrates Resistance Band Curls

Benefits

Both your back and biceps play a pivotal role in your daily life. From pulling to pushing to lifting, these two muscle groups are necessary for practical strength and a shredded upper body. As you grow older, things get heavier due to the body's decline. Some benefits of exercising the back and biceps are listed below.

1. Improved strength – This benefit is evident in the lives of seniors who actively engage these muscles during exercise. It strengthens the muscles in your arms, enabling you to carry items more effortlessly, take things down from elevated shelves, and even put up yourself out of an armchair more comfortably. You engage easily in your everyday activities, opening doors, lifting laundry baskets, or even turning open a stuck jar.

2. Better mobility – if you regularly engage in back and bicep exercises, your shoulders, elbows, or wrists won't be tight. This workout will stretch and strengthen your arms and help alleviate discomfort, avoid muscle loss and keep you working as smoothly as possible.

3. Reduces the chance of injury – As you grow older, your body can become weaker and more vulnerable to injury. By engaging in this workout, your joints and muscles' strength will improve, and they'll be thicker and less liable to be injured. A strong back helps keep your body's posture correct and can prevent injuries from improper movement.

4. Toning and shaping – These exercises can help fix tone up flabby arms or even help with weight loss goals. It keeps overweight seniors in shape and tones up muscles needed for daily activities. Exercising the back and biceps will build and maintain strong back and bicep muscles.

The advantages of exercising the back and the bicep together cannot be overemphasized. To enjoy your golden years, integrate these exercises into your daily workout routine and watch strength and flexibility surge back into your body.

Chapter 5 Work Your Chest and Triceps

The chest and triceps are two more fundamental muscle groups that can be exercised together. The chest is the primary and larger muscle group in this pairing. At the same time, the triceps are the supplemental source of power.

The chest and triceps are also known as the "push" muscles. They are used for moving things like a chair away from the body or moving the body away from an object like the floor. The workout's focus should begin with the larger muscle focus and usually the most challenging movement or the exercise that requires the most strength. Depending on how you feel, this may be the best course of action. If you are not feeling up to some of the more difficult moves, it is okay to skip them and focus on getting a workout by using less intense exercises.

Working out these two muscle groups together instead of splitting them up can help maximize time and open the opportunity for a rest day or some other exercise-focused day. For example, suppose you wanted to do more cardio days. In that case, you could make sure to combine chest and triceps, back and biceps so that you'll have an extra day when you're ready for cardio. It can also help provide extra weight for the smaller triceps to help push as the chest does most of the work.

These exercises are just another tool in your inventory to make life better as a senior. Focus on engaging the chest and triceps (on the back of the arm, opposite the biceps) to build strength and stability while ensuring you are doing what you can to maintain your independence.

Examples of workouts in this category are:

Pushups: This traditional exercise uses your chest and triceps to lift or move your body away from a stationary surface like the floor or wall.

Overhead Dumbbell Press: This exercise uses the upper body. It focuses on strengthening the shoulders while using the chest and triceps as support.

Bench Press- The bench press requires you to lie down on a surface and push dumbbells or a barbell away from the body using the chest and triceps.

Home Workout for Chest and Triceps with No Equipment

These at-home exercises should be easy to complete with little planning other than a warm-up. For these, you will just need some basic items you can find in most locations where you would be working out. These exercises will help strengthen the chest and triceps.

Wall Pushup

1. Stand next to a wall or stationary flat surface where you can place your arms slightly wider than shoulder length apart.

2. Move your feet back away from the wall and keep them about shoulder length apart. Keep your arms extended at about shoulder height with palms flat on the wall. Keep your body at a comfortable angle with feet flat on the ground.

3. Inhale. Engage your core and slowly lower your body towards the wall by bending at the elbows. Your feet should remain planted, and your legs and back should all remain as in line as possible.

4. Exhale and use your chest and arms to press yourself back until your arms are fully extended once again. This is one

repetition.

5. Repeat this movement for two sets of 8-10 repetitions. Rest 30-60 seconds between sets.

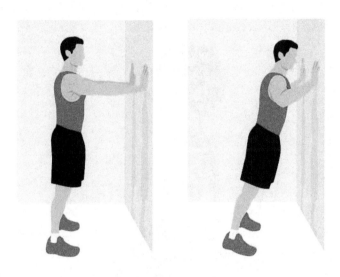

51. A man demonstrates a wall pushup.

Chair Dips

Note: For this exercise, you'll need a chair; for beginners or those with strength restrictions, it will require a chair with arms. Make sure to get a sturdy chair that is not going to move.

1. With feet slightly less than shoulder-width apart, stand in front of a securely planted chair as if you're about to sit. Reach back and grasp the arms of the chair with your hands and sit in the chair.

2. Bend at the elbows as you grasp the arms of the chair. Your feet should be planted on the floor in front of you, and your knees will be bent. Keep your chest up, back straight, and neck neutral. Exhale. Push off the arms of the chair using

your triceps and chest. Raise yourself up and out of the chair. Do not lock your elbows.

3. Inhale and lower yourself back down into the chair. When lowered into the chair, your elbows should go out and back behind you. Only lift yourself as high as you feel comfortable regarding your elbows and shoulders.

4. Repeat this movement for three sets of 10-12 repetitions. Rest 30-60 seconds between sets.

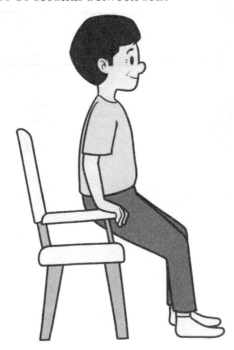

52. A man performs chair dips using chair arms for support.

Pushup

This exercise can be done on the floor with legs extended or on the floor with knees down instead to make it easier.

1. Lie face down on the ground with legs extended. Place hands on either side of the body slightly wider than shoulder length apart. Palms should be down on the floor right below shoulder level.

2. Engage core to help keep the back straight. Keep your neck neutral as you look down at the floor below you. Exhale and press up using the triceps and chest until the body comes up off the ground. Lift the body up until the arms are fully extended. Pause for a second at the top of the movement.

Modification: If performing this exercise from the knees, keep your back straight, and extend your arms when pressing. The knees will remain together and planted on the ground throughout the movement. Lower legs can either be held together off the ground the entire movement or lay still together on the ground.

3. Inhale and slowly lower your body back down to the ground.

4. Repeat this movement for three sets of 10 repetitions. Rest for 60 seconds between sets.

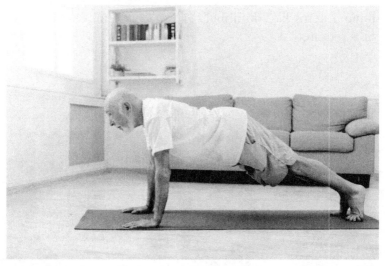

53. A senior performs a pushup.

Incline Pushup

1. Find a surface about the same height as a kitchen counter. Grasp the edges of the counter with hands slightly wider than shoulder length apart.

2. Move your feet back from the counter until your arms are almost fully extended. Keep feet slightly apart for balance. Keep your back, neck, and legs straight throughout the movement.

3. Inhale and lower yourself down until your elbows are at about a 90-degree angle, if possible. Engage your core.

4. Exhale and use your chest and triceps to press your body up and back until your arms are almost fully extended again. Your heels may come up slightly during this movement but try to keep them from moving too much.

5. Repeat this exercise for two sets of 8-10 repetitions. Rest for 60 seconds between sets.

Home Workout for Back and Biceps with Equipment

For these exercises, you will need some basic exercise equipment. Most of the items can now be purchased at local big box stores or online. Sporting goods stores will also carry this equipment, though they may not be located near your area. Some of these exercises can also be completed with household objects as a substitute if items like dumbbells haven't been purchased or lighter weight is required.

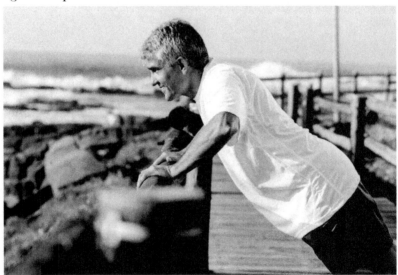

54. A man performs an incline pushup.

Floor Bench Press

1. Grab a set of dumbbells or a barbell and find an open area where you can lack face up on the floor. Keep one dumbbell on each side of the body or grasp the barbell with hands wider than shoulder length apart.

2. Your elbows and triceps will begin the movement on the floor. Bend your knees and keep your feet planted on the floor. Your back should remain flat and neck neutral as you look up at the ceiling above you. The bar or dumbbells should be at your chest line.

3. Exhale. Press the dumbbells or barbell away from your body using your chest and triceps until your arms are extended in front of you.

4. Inhale. Slowly lower the bar down to the starting position with triceps on the floor.

5. Repeat this movement for three sets of 10 repetitions. Rest for 30-60 seconds between sets.

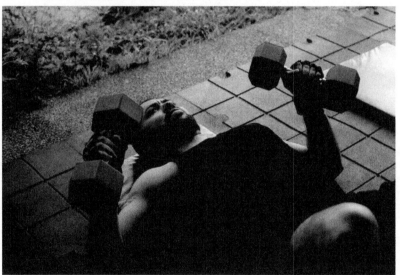

55. A man performs a bench press on the floor.

Overhead Press

Option: This exercise can be done seated in a secure chair or standing. This exercise can be completed with a barbell or dumbbells. If the weight is too heavy, this exercise can be completed with something lighter like water bottles or apples in hand.

1. Grab a set of dumbbells or alternative weight. Stand tall with feet shoulder-width apart. Engage the core.

2. Lift dumbbells up to shoulder height by bending elbows. Hands and dumbbells should be slightly out in front of the shoulders. Keep the back straight and neck neutral.

3. Exhale, and using the shoulders, press the dumbbells up overhead. Press them until arms are extended, but do not lock out elbows.

4. Inhale and slowly lower the dumbbells back to about shoulder height.

5. Repeat this exercise for three sets for 8-10 repetitions. Rest for 60 seconds between sets.

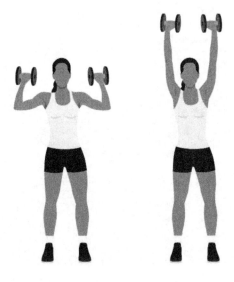

56. A woman demonstrating the overhead press.

Triceps Extension

Note: This exercise can be completed from a standing or seated position. It can also be completed with one arm at a time using lighter weights or both arms together on a single slightly heavier weight.

1. Sit in a sturdy chair that allows clearance to move the arms around the upper body and overhead. Keep a straight back and neck. Engage the core to hold the body upright. Grab a light dumbbell.

2. Hold the weight by the back of your head. Your elbow will be bent, and your palm will be facing toward your head.

3. Exhale and use your triceps to extend the arm until it is fully extended overhead.

4. Inhale and slowly lower the weight back down beside your head.

5. Repeat this exercise for three sets of 10-12 repetitions. Rest for 30-60 seconds between sets.

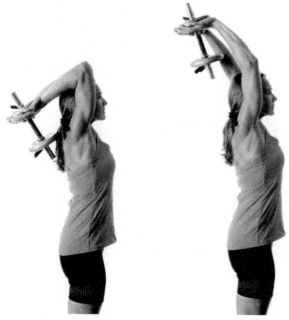

57. A woman demonstrates the triceps extension

Chest Fly

Note: This exercise can be completed on an exercise bench for a greater stretch, but it is safer lying flat on the ground.

1. Grab a pair of dumbbells and lie face up on the ground. Bend your knees and keep your feet planted on the floor.

2. Raise the dumbbells until they are outstretched in front of you at chest length. Palms will be facing inward toward each other. Keep a very slight bend at the elbow.

3. Inhale and slowly lower the dumbbells down to your sides. This movement will open the chest and form a "T" on the ground with your arms and torso. Stop lowering once the triceps portions of your upper arms touch the ground.

4. Exhale, and using your chest, pull your extended arms back up and out in front of you to the starting position.

5. Repeat this movement for two sets of 10-12 reps

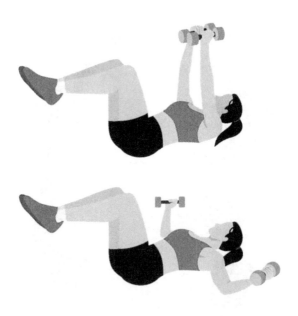

58. A woman demonstrates a dumbbell chest fly on the floor.

Gym Workout for Chest and Triceps

These exercises can be performed at most gyms. They use basic gym machines, which are often the safest way for older adults to perform some exercises. There is often more than one machine that can be used to perform the same movement. Be sure to read the instructions on the exercise machine for guidance on what muscle you'll be working and the proper use of the machine.

Seated Chest Press Machine

Note: Look for the machine with the tall and narrow chair for upright seating with the arms and handles out in front of the machine.

1. Adjust the weight pin on the machine to a suitable weight for you. It is always better to start low and work your way up for safety.

2. Sit down in the chair with your back firmly against it. Make sure the handles for the machine are sitting at chest height to you while seated. Plant feet firmly on the floor in front of you.

3. Grasp the handles so your elbows are bent by your side or slightly behind you. Exhale, and using your chest and triceps, press the handles outward until your arms are fully extended. Hands will end up in a raised position slightly closer together than the start position.

4. Inhale and slowly lower the handles back down to the starting position.

5. Perform this movement for three sets of 10 reps. Rest for 3-60 seconds between sets.

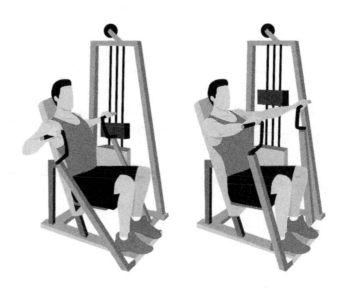

59. A man demonstrating the chest press machine

Smith Machine Bench Press

Note: The Smith machine is a version of a standard bench that provides a guided barbell line for the weight to travel upon. It also provides moveable safety guards on the machine so that if weight is dropped, the exerciser is protected. Be sure to test out the safety features and ensure they are in place before attempting this exercise.

1. Position a weight bench perpendicularly under the barbell of the Smith machine. Ensure it is in the center of the machine. Test the bar positioning by lying on the bench under the secure and unweighted bar to ensure the bar lands at chest height when lowered.

2. Ensure the stop pads located below where the weight is placed on the bar are at a suitable height. For safety, put them higher than the bench and at a height where the bar is stopped by it before getting close to your chest at its lowest.

3. Lower the bar so it is high enough above the bench so you can lie down and slide into the proper position. Add weight to the outsides of the barbell connected to the Smith machine. Slide weights off the stationary racks on the machine and then slide them onto the moveable bar. Be sure to keep even weight on both sides. Start with a lower weight as the amount can always be increased.

   Note: It is recommended to try this exercise with no weight first to ensure the angles are correct.

5. Get in position under the bar and grasp the bar with arms wider than shoulder length apart. Your head, back, and buttocks will all be flat on the bench, while your legs will be on either side. Plant your feet on the floor.

6. Grip the bar and turn it so the hooks unclasp from the machine freeing the bar. Exhale, and using your chest and triceps, press the bar up and away from your chest. Raise it until your arms are almost fully extended.

6. Inhale and slowly lower the bar back down. To rack the bar, simply turn your wrists and re-hook the bar to the machine.

7. Perform this exercise for three sets of 10 repetitions. Rest for 60 seconds after each set.

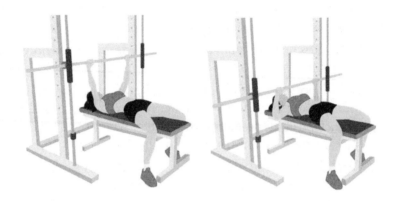

60. A woman demonstrating the Smith machine bench press.

Triceps Cable Pushdown

Option: Multiple handles can be attached and used for this exercise. The most common two would be the straight bar or the short rope with the balls on the ends.

1. Find the cable extension machine you can stand in front of with the adjustable "tree." Adjust the cable height on the machine so it is at the top of the machine/tree. Attach the short rope handle with the balls on the end of either side of the rope.

2. Adjust the weight so that it is right for you. Step back slightly from the machine so there is room in front of you. Reach up and grab the rope handles. Keep your feet together and planted flat on the floor. Keep your back straight and your neck neutral.

3. Pull the cable down and towards your body until your elbows are at a 90-degree angle. Exhale. Using your triceps push the cable handle down while spreading your hands apart. Your upper arms should stay right by your sides as you bend only at the elbow. The balls of the cable will end up on either side of your thigh as your hands will be by your pockets

4. Inhale and slowly let the cable raise back up until your arms are at a 90-degree angle.

5. Perform this movement for three sets of 10 repetitions with 30-60 seconds of rest between sets.

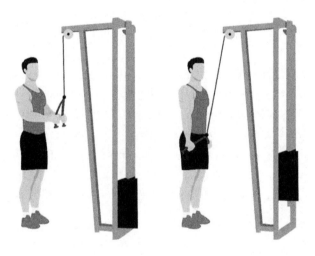

61. A man demonstrates the triceps cable pushdown

Shoulder Press Machine

Note: This machine performs the same movement as the Overhead Shoulder Press. This can be used as a substitute or to help beginners build a foundation for the movement. There are also two different grip variations on the handles: one with palms facing inward and one with palms facing forward. Either grip can be used and will still exercise the shoulders.

1. Find the shoulder press machine. It will have a long skinny chair for sitting upright, and the arms and handles will be in the air on either side of the head. Adjust the weight using the pin so that it is light enough for you to press overhead comfortably.

2. Adjust the bottom of the seat so that it is low enough, and you can grab the handles with your elbows at a 90-degree angle. This should be the bottom and starting position of the movement.

3. Keep your back straight against the seat. Keep your neck neutral and head back against the seat back. Your feet will be spread apart and planted on the ground in front of you on either side of the seat.

4. Grasp the bar so your palms are facing forward. Keep your wrists straight. Your elbows should be slightly in front of your body. Start from a 90-degree angle and maintain a slight bend in the elbow throughout. Your elbows should stay in line with your hips. Engage your core.

5. Exhale. Press the bars straight over your head until your arms are almost fully extended.

6. Inhale and lower the bars until your elbow reaches 90 degrees.

7. Perform this movement for three sets of 8-10 repetitions.

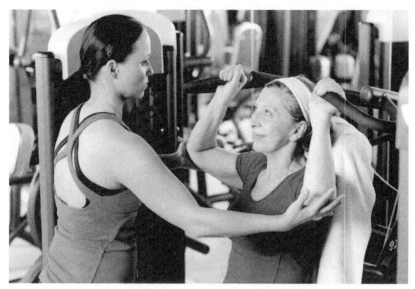
62. A woman uses the shoulder press machine.

Partner Workout for Chest and Triceps

These workouts are made to be completed with a partner. The partner will serve as support, and exercisers take turns, or the moves can be performed together. Encourage one another to keep going and stay dedicated to the workout. Keep a watchful eye and/or ear (if performing alongside) on your partner to ensure they are safe during the exercises. Partner workouts should be a social activity. The other exercises listed can be done with a partner for support or by taking turns performing the exercise. These exercises will require at least one resistance band.

Triceps Kickback

1. The first partner will be the anchor and should grab a resistance band and hold it tightly at about chest level in front of them. The other partner should face this partner and grab the other end of the resistance band in one hand. Step back until the band is almost taut.

2. The second partner should keep feet slightly less than shoulder-width apart. Bend at the waist until the upper body creates a 45-degree angle. Keep the upper part of the arm in line with the upper body.

3. Keep the back straight. Your elbow should begin at a 90-degree angle with the band in front of the body. Exhale. Using the triceps extend the arm back until the elbow is straight.

4. Inhale and allow the elbow to return to the 90-degree angle.

5. Repeat this movement for two sets of 8-10 repetitions. Rest 30-60 seconds between sets.

6. Switch sides and let the anchor partner perform the exercise.

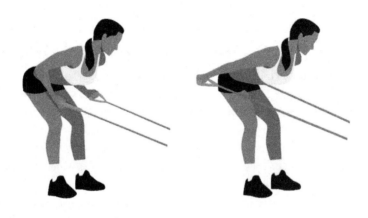

63. A woman demonstrates the resistance band triceps kickback.

Cable Press

Note: For this exercise, choose a cable that's big enough and flexible enough for both partners to be able to fulfill their parts. One partner will act as an anchor while the other presses the resistance band.

1. Partner 1 will stand behind partner 2 and serve as the anchor by holding a resistance band. Partner two will grab the ends of the resistance band and take a small step away from their partner.

2. Feet should be planted with a wide stance for the anchor, and the cable will be held in both hands just under chest level. Partner two will step one foot in front of the other for a sturdier stance.

3. Partner two will position arms at chest height on either side of the body while grasping handles. Palms will be facing down. Engage the core. Partner two will exhale and use the chest and triceps to press the cable in front of their body. Partner one will hold tight and engage the core to keep from moving. Hands will end up closer together, and arms will be fully at the end of the move.

4. Partner two will breathe and allow arms to come back into the starting position with elbows at 90-degree angles.

5. Repeat this movement for three sets of 10 reps. Rest 30-60 seconds between sets. Switch after completing all sets or in between sets so partners can take turns.

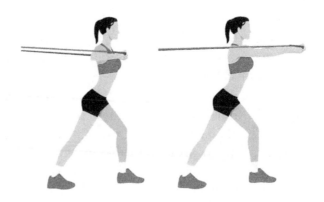

64. A woman performs a resistance band cable press.

Partner Pushups

This exercise is a basic pushup that can be performed against the wall, on the ground, or at an incline on a kitchen counter. Partners can either try to perform their complete set first or see who can reach the entire set and rep suggestions.

Modification: This exercise can be done on the knees or with legs fully extended, depending on your fitness level.

1. Partners should find an open space where both can perform the pushups side by side or face one another.

2. Partners should lie face down on the ground with palms at chest height. Hands should be positioned wider than shoulder length apart on the ground. Elbows will be bent at the start of this exercise. The back should be kept straight, and the neck will remain neutral as you look at the floor below you.

3. Both partners should count aloud as they perform repetitions. Exhale and press up using your chest and triceps to raise your body off the ground. If using knees, everything

about the knees should be raised off the ground. Press up until arms are almost fully extended.

4. Inhale and slowly lower back down to the starting position.

5. Repeat this movement for three sets of 10 reps. Rest for 60 seconds between sets. Partners should strive to complete movement with proper form.

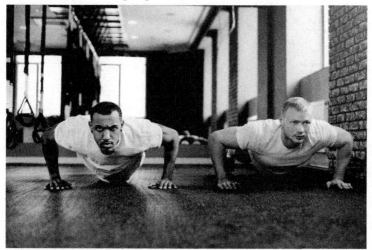

65. Partners perform pushups together

Chest and Triceps Workout Benefits

As seniors, exercising your chest and triceps is crucial. Keeping the chest strong will help balance the body and even out strength. The triceps perform tasks such as pulling open a dishwasher door or getting up from a chair. Exercising the chest and triceps will provide pushing power.

Benefits:

1. Strength

Keeping the chest and triceps strong allows older adults to help maintain their independence. A strong chest can help you pick yourself up off the ground, and your triceps can help lift yourself out of a seat or sit up in bed. Having a strong chest will be important when it comes to many daily tasks. Pushing power is a part of everyday life.

2. Reduce Injury

By maintaining pushing power, you can ensure that you are in a better position to handle the encounter of daily life. You don't want to get into a position where you try to move a chair or get up from a seat and fall. Keeping a strong chest and triceps will help protect your joints from taking the brunt of a movement and possibly becoming injured

3. Aesthetics

Exercising the chest can help add to the size and look of the upper body. Men who want a bigger-looking upper body will benefit from strengthening the chest. Women who want an hourglass figure with a strong upper body will benefit from chest workouts.

Exercising the triceps will help keep the arms looking strong and toned. In a short-sleeved or sleeveless top, a well-defined triceps muscle always looks exceptionally good for men and women.

Exercising the triceps and chest will help you to reach your arm goals and may be able to replace flab with muscle.

4. Shoulder Stability

Shoulders are an essential part of the pushing power of the body and are therefore grouped with the chest and triceps. Keeping strong shoulders will help prevent injury. You use your shoulders more than you think, and it is important to maintain a sturdy shoulder to protect the joint there.

Shoulder strength can help reach overhead to grab something from a cabinet or remove a shirt overhead.

Disclaimer:

If you have had any previous issues or pains in your chest, seek medical advice before engaging in chest exercises. Once you have been verified to be fit, avoid lifting overly heavy objects or the ones. Be aware of the danger of pressing weights over the body, including the chest and head.

Chapter 6 Work Your Legs

The legs are a crucial part of the body for a senior to maintain independence. The legs offer a lot of challenges and trouble for older adults. They, therefore, need to receive extra close attention when exercising.

The legs help keep you mobile. If they are injured or too weak to support you safely, suddenly you can't participate in many activities. The legs need to be kept strong to preserve your ability to move around the house. The legs help us bend over to pick things up, move across a room, and get out of a chair.

Keeping the legs strong can help prevent falls and make you feel more stable when walking or bending over. These exercises are usually straightforward and very functional; the goal is to build power in the legs. Many leg exercises also incorporate other body parts, which can be taxing.

Be sure to warm up well before leg workouts to reduce the risk of falling or injuring a joint. Leg exercises are meant to keep you going, not keep you sidelined. Be aware of your limitations as you perform these valuable exercises.

Some examples of leg exercises include:

Squat: The body lowers itself down, bending at the waist and knees. This move simulates squatting down without bending over to pick something off the floor.

Step-Ups: This exercise helps keep the leg muscles strong as you lift your body up onto the next step using your leg muscles.

Stationary Bicycle: The bicycle can serve as an excellent workout for the legs. It requires an extensive range of motion and can require strength to push through the resistance.

Home Workout for Legs with No Equipment

These workouts will only require a standard chair to perform, and they can mostly be done anywhere and require little else besides a warm-up.

Chair Squat

Modification: The squat is an integral part of any exercise routine. For this exercise, you will use a chair with or without arms (the arms can assist with progression). However, it can be done standing behind a chair and holding the back for support or without a chair.

1. Find a chair that is not too deep-set. You'll want to be able to get up using just your legs and buttocks. Sit in the chair, so your feet are planted firmly on the ground in front of you, slightly wider than hip-width apart. Scoot forward if necessary to achieve this position. Your knees should be at about a 90-degree angle.

2. Keep your back straight and your neck neutral. Bend forwards a little from the hips. You can cross your arms over your chest, extend your arms straight out in front of you, or use the arms of the chair to help you until further strength is achieved. Exhale and straighten your knees and hips to get up from the chair. Press forward through your hips and up through your feet. You should end straight up right in front of the chair.

3. Inhale and slowly lower yourself down and back into the chair until your knees and feet are in the starting position again.

4. Repeat this movement for three sets of 12 repetitions. Rest for 60 seconds between sets.

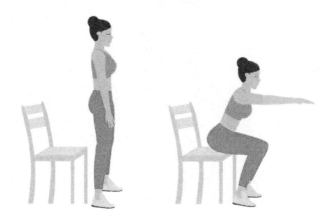

66. A woman performs a chair squat.

Standing Leg Raises

1. Stand up straight beside a wall, chair, or kitchen counter for balance support. Place one arm on the back of the chair if necessary for balance.

2. Engage your core to help maintain balance. Exhale. Lift your right leg off the ground until you create a 90-degree angle with your knee. The thigh should end up parallel to the ground. Keep the other foot planted on the floor with the leg straight. Pause for a second at the top.

3. Inhale. Slowly lower your foot back down to the ground.

4. Repeat this movement for each leg for three sets of 8-10 repetitions. Rest for 30-60 seconds between sets.

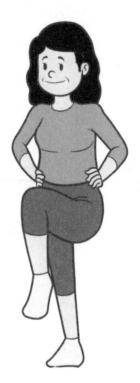

67. Women perform standing leg raises without holding support.

Floor Bridge

1. Lie on the ground face up. Bend your knees so your feet are planted flat on the ground about hip-width apart. Extend your arms and place your hand palms down on the ground beside your body.

2. Keep a neutral neck. Engage your core and exhale. Push through your feet and squeeze your buttocks (also known as glutes) to raise your buttocks and lower back up off the floor. Press up through your hips. Your thighs and body will form a straight line, and your knees will be at a 90-degree angle at the top of this movement. The top of your back, shoulders, feet, and head will remain on the ground.

3. Inhale as you lower back down into the starting position. Your back and buttocks should be on the floor and your knees back to a smaller angle.

4. Repeat this movement for three sets of 10-12 reps. Rest for 30-60 seconds between sets.

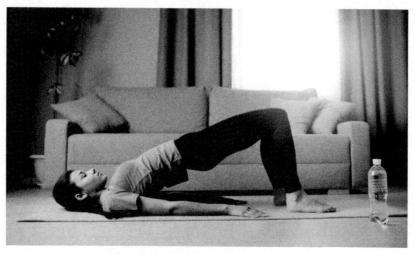

68. A young lady performing a floor bridge.

Knee Extensions

1. Sit in a chair or couch high enough so the knees can sit at a 90-degree angle with feet planted on the floor directly below the knees. Move around in the chair if necessary to achieve a position where the chair supports the thighs.

2. Sit up straight in the chair with your chest up and shoulders back. Maintain a neutral neck. Place hands over thighs for support. Exhale. Extend left leg at the knee. Raise the lower part of the leg until it forms a straight line with the rest of the leg parallel to the floor.

3. Inhale and slowly lower the leg back down to the 90-degree angle starting position.

4. Repeat this movement for three sets of 10 repetitions for each leg. Rest for 30-60 seconds between sets.

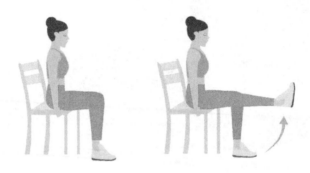

69. A woman demonstrates a seated knee extension.

Home Workout for Legs with Equipment

These exercises will require some basic exercise equipment that can be used at home or most places you would work out. These items can be purchased at sports stores, many big box stores, and online. If you haven't purchased the specific equipment, other substitute weights or objects from around the house can be used. For these exercises, you will likely need a pair of dumbbells and a step platform.

Step-ups

For this exercise, you will need a step platform or another safe flat surface to step up on. A porch step could be used if it is in a safe spot and is not too high.

Note: This exercise can be done from multiple angles to help improve balance on strength when moving or stepping in various directions. You can step on and back off, on and over, laterally(sidestep) on and off, or laterally up and over. You can also begin on the step and step down and back up. Use these different angles to make the workout more challenging or to keep the workout exciting.

1. Stand in front of the step. The feet should only be slightly apart. Pay attention to where the step is in front of you.

2. Exhale and lead with the right foot; step up onto the step.

3. Follow through by bringing the left foot up onto the step. The step should be a fluid 1-2 movement.

4. Inhale and step off of the step, leading with your right foot. Follow through with the left.

5. Repeat this movement for three sets of 10-12 reps. Switch legs and lead with the left foot first for another three sets. Rest for 60 seconds between sets.

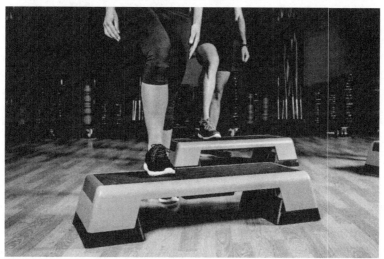

70. A man and woman using a step-up platform.

Calf Raises

Depending on your fitness level, for this exercise, you will need a chair for support, no equipment, or a set of light dumbbells. You can begin by using the chair and progress to the dumbbells.

1. Stand with light dumbbells in your hands by your sides. Keep feet close together.

2. Exhale and push up through the balls of your feet. Use your calves to raise your mid feet and heels off the ground. Move slowly and do not bounce.

3. Breathe out and slowly lower yourself down. Once your feet are flat on the ground, lean slightly back on your heels to raise your toes and balls of your feet off the ground.

4. Return to flat foot briefly before repeating the movement from the beginning.

5. Repeat for two sets of 10 repetitions. Rest for 30-60 seconds between sets.

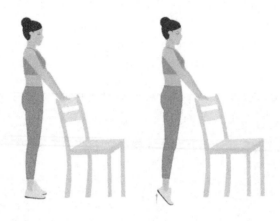

71. A woman demonstrates calf raises.

Hip Marching

For this exercise, you will need a chair and ankle weights.

1. Sit in a sturdy chair with feet on the floor. Keep your back straight and neck neutral.

2. Keep hands on thighs for support. Engage your core for stability. Exhale as you lift your right leg as high as possible while maintaining a 90-degree bend in the knee. Pause for a second at the top.

3. Inhale and lower your leg back down to the floor.

4. Switch legs and repeat the movement.

5. Do two sets of 10 reps for each leg. Rest 30-60 seconds between sets.

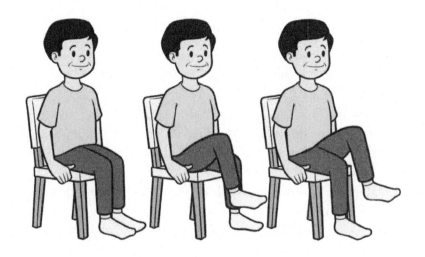

72. An older man performing hip marching in a chair

Deadlift

The Deadlift is a great exercise that uses many muscles of the body at the same time. It is especially useful for strengthening the back and legs. Use deadlifts as a powerful leg exercise but be careful when performing it on the same day as squats as they are both very taxing.

Option: This exercise can be done with s set of dumbbells, a barbell, or something with some weight that can be gripped from around the house, such as a loaded backpack or laundry basket.

1. Stand tall with chest up and feet shoulder-width apart. Shoulders should be pulled back; there should be a slight arch in the back.

2. Dumbbells should begin in your hands in front of your thighs with palms facing towards the body.

3. Bend down by hinging at the hip and bending the knees. The back should be kept straight (don't let it round), and the neck should be in a neutral position with eyes looking in front of you.

4. Keeping arms straight, lower the dumbbells down right in front of your legs as you hinge your hips and bend your knees. If you can get your upper body down to parallel, that's great, but otherwise, just lower until you feel the stretch in your lower back and hamstrings.

5. Pull the weights up by thrusting your hips forward to their natural position and pushing up through your feet. You should end up in an upright standing position with the weights in front of your thighs.

6. Repeat for three sets of 8 reps with 60 seconds of rest between sets.

NOTE: Start with a lighter weight and progress to heavier once a foundation of strength and balance has been built for this movement.

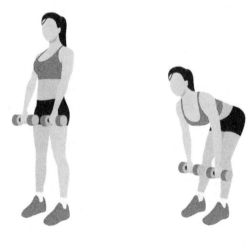

73. A woman is performing a dumbbell Deadlift.

Gym Workout for Legs

These exercises will be completed in a gym setting where there are leg machines available. The leg machines at the gym are a great option to perform similar alternatives to many of the exercises listed in the previous leg sections.

Leg Press

1. Find the leg press machine with the seat and square platform perpendicular to the ground for your feet. Adjust the platform and seat so that you can sit up straight with chest out and legs at a 90-degree angle as they rest flat on the platform in front of you.

2. Adjust the weight so it's challenging but not overwhelming. Engage the core. Exhale and push out through your legs to extend them and move the platform away from your body. Do not lock your knees.

3. Inhale. Slowly return your legs to the starting 90-degree angle position.

4. Perform this movement for two sets of 8-10 repetitions. Rest for 60 seconds between sets.

GYM WORKOUT
Leg Press

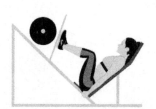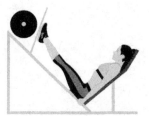

74. A woman using a leg press machine.

Leg Extension Machine

1. Find the leg extension machine with a seat that may have padded bars over the thighs to secure you and another

padded bar below them for your shins.

2. Adjust the seat's back so your legs adequately fit in the pads at the bottom of your shins. Adjust the shin pad so that it's almost right below the edge of the seat. Be sure to check all the adjustments so the movement feels comfortable. The weight and work from the exercise should be put on the quadriceps or muscle on the top of the thigh. The exercise should not strain your knee joint. If there are hand grips by the seat, use them to hold you in place and remove strain on the back of the knees.

3. Adjust the weight so that it's right for you. Slip your shins behind the pad so that extending legs will raise it forward. Engage the core. Exhale and push the padded bar out with your legs using the muscle on the top of the thigh. Extend your knees so that your legs are almost fully extended into a straight line.

4. Inhale and slowly lower the padded bar to almost the starting position.

5. Repeat this exercise for three sets of 10 repetitions. Rest for 30-60 seconds between sets.

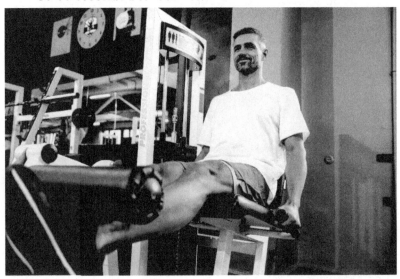

75. A senior using the leg extension machine

Seated Leg Curl Machine

1. Find the leg curl machine. It will have a chair with a back, a padded bar that looks like a leg rest out in front of the seat, and a bar with handles where the steering wheel would go.

2. Sit in the machine and put your legs up and on top of the padded bar in front of you. Adjust the back of the seat so that you're close enough to the bar to pull it down with the back of your calves. You can also adjust the height of the padded bar for comfort so it hits the right spot- towards the bottom of your calves. Legs should be almost fully extended on top of the pad to be in the proper position when starting.

3. Lower the thigh restraint onto the top of the thighs to snugly hold down your legs. Grip the handles above the restraint bar to hold yourself in place.

4. Exhale. Contracting the hamstrings (on the back of the thigh), pull the padded bar back towards the seat with the back of your legs. Stop when you feel the stretch on the top of your thigh or when you hit a 90-degree angle with your knee.

5. Inhale and let your legs extend back out.

6. Perform this exercise for two to three sets of 10 repetitions with 60 seconds of rest between sets.

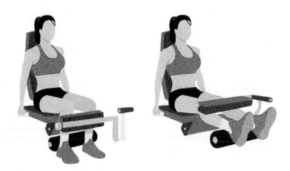

76. A woman demonstrates the leg curl machine.

Seated Calf Raise Machine

1. Find the seated calf raise machine. It will have a seat with no back or arms and a pad to secure over the thighs. In front of the seat will be the arms with the weights.

1. Adjust the weight on the machine using free weights if necessary. Be sure to start with lighter weights until you have built flexibility up for this movement.

2. Sit in the seat and put your toes on the edge of the platform steps. These will be located near the ground and in front of the seat. Lower the thigh restraint down on top of the thighs to hold them in place.

3. Raise your heels to lift the weights and unlock the machine. Grab the handle by your knee while raising the weight and move it in towards the weights. The weight will now rest on your thighs and be held up under your own power.

4. Keep your knees at a 90-degree angle and keep your back straight and chest up.

5. Inhale and lower your heels down to below your toe level if possible. You should feel a stretch in the calves and near the ankle, but it shouldn't be painful.

6. Exhale and use the calves to raise heels up and push the bar on the thighs upward. Keep your toes on the steps. Lift weight as high as possible by pushing the heels above the toes and step level. To leave the machine, raise your heel and push the lever by your knees out to the side to lock the weights in place. You may now exit the machine

7. Perform this exercise for two sets of 10 reps with 30-60 seconds of rest between sets.

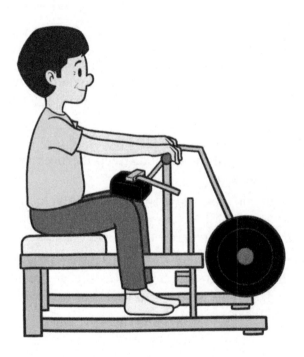

77. A man using the seated calf raise machine.

Partner Workout for Legs

These workouts should be done with a partner and can be completed at home or anywhere with some basic equipment, including a step platform and chairs. The goal of these workouts is to have motivational support while using your partner as a safety precaution when performing challenging movements.

Partner Lunge

This exercise can either be done with two partners and chairs performing the exercise simultaneously while facing each other or with partners taking turns and providing support to the other's hand during the motion.

1. Get a sturdy chair. Stand with your left side to the back of the chair. Grab the top of the chair for support with your left hand. A partner can serve as support for the right hand. The support partner would stand with legs hip-width apart, facing the exercising partner. Put hands together at about the same height as the chair back to form secondary support for the lunger to grab.

2. Step back with your right leg until it is at about a 45-degree angle. The front leg should be planted firmly with the knee bent as well. Keep your back straight and head up.

3. Inhale and dip down, bending at the knees. The front and back knees should be as close to 90 degrees as possible. Keep the front foot planted flat. The toes of the back foot will remain on the ground. Keep the back close to straight under the body.

4. Exhale and push up through the feet to raise the body up and out of the lunge. Use the chair back and a partner for support until your strength is built.

5. Perform this exercise for three sets of 8 reps and rest for 60 seconds between sets. Switch legs after the first three sets are complete. Partners can also take turns switching positions between sets.

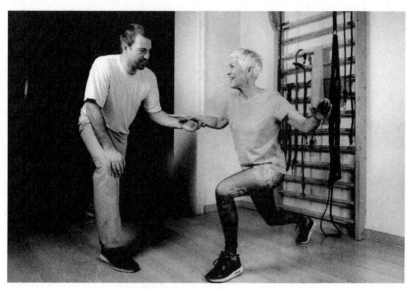

78. A senior performs a lunge with a partner

Partner Step-Ups

You will need a step platform or a wide step that isn't too tall for this exercise.

1. Place the step platform in an open, secure place on the ground.

2. Partners should stand on either side of the platform facing each other.

3. Partner 1 should exhale and, leading with the right foot, step up onto the platform. The left foot should step onto the platform secondly.

4. Partner 1 should inhale and step back down, leading with the right foot first. Partners should remain facing each other throughout the exercise.

5. Partner 2 should exhale and step onto the platform leading with their right foot. The left foot should follow.

6. Partner 2 will inhale and step back off the platform, leading with the right foot first.

7. Partners will take turns going up and down the steps. Perform this exercise for two sets of 10-12 reps for each leg. Rest for 30 seconds between sets.

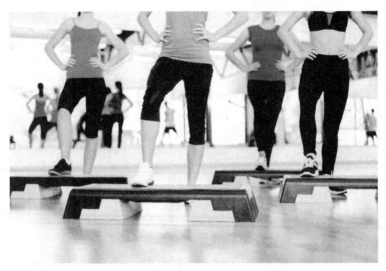

79. Young adults perform step-ups together

Partner Chair Squats

This exercise will require a sturdy chair. Partners can either serve as support to help one another perform the squat, or two chairs can be used, and partners can perform the squats together.

1. Find a chair that is not too deep-set. You'll want to be able to get up using just your legs and buttocks. Sit in the chair, so your feet are planted firmly on the ground in front of you, slightly wider than hip-width apart. Scoot forward if necessary to achieve this position. Your knees should be at about a 90-degree angle.

2. Partner 2 can stand a step in front of you with elbows bent to close to 90-degree angles with palms up for support.

3. Partner 1, you should keep your back straight and your neck neutral. Bend forwards a little from the hips. Reach your arms straight out in front of you. Exhale and straighten out your knees and hips to get up out of the chair. Press forward through your hips and up through your feet. As you rise, if need be, use Partner 2's hands for support to complete the movement. You should end up standing straight up right in front of the chair, facing your partner.

4. Inhale and slowly lower yourself down and back into the chair until your knees and feet are in the starting position again.

5. Repeat this movement for three sets of 12 repetitions. Rest for 60 seconds between sets. Partners can alternate sets of squatting and supporting.

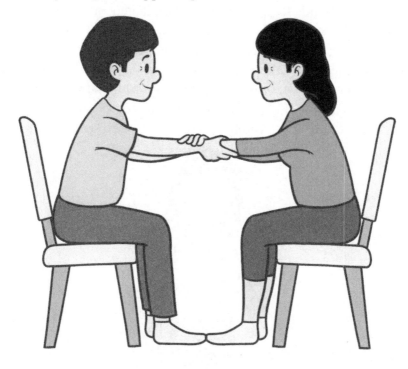

80. Partners assist each other with the chair squat

Leg Lifts Partner

This exercise increases balance, core stability, and leg strength by using a partner to assist as a supporter if necessary. If partners don't need support, two chairs can be used, and the move can be performed simultaneously while facing one another.

1. Partners should stand up straight beside a wall, chair, or kitchen counter for balance support. If possible, turn the support so partners can face one another and stand relatively close. Place one arm on the back of the support if necessary for balance. The other arm can go on a partner if necessary for support.

2. Engage your cores to help maintain balance. Exhale. Lift your right leg off the ground until you create a 90-degree angle with your knee. The thigh should end up parallel to the ground. Keep the other foot planted on the floor with the leg straight. Pause for a second at the top.

3. Inhale. Slowly lower your foot back down to the ground. Partners can take turns with one raising their leg while the other lowers it, or they can raise them simultaneously

4. Repeat this movement for each leg for three sets of 8-10 repetitions. Rest for 30-60 seconds between sets.

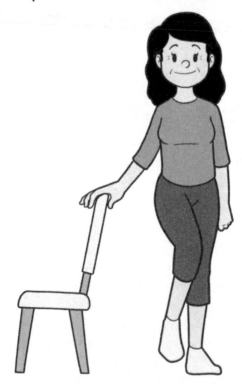

81. A woman performs a standing leg lift with a chair

Leg Workout Benefits

Everyone needs to have strong legs. The legs are the motor that keeps you moving around. Seniors need to exercise their legs as it gets harder to maintain joints and muscles as they age. Exercising the legs can increase power, confidence, and mobility.

Benefits:

1. Strength

Having strong legs means being able to get up out of the chair or off the ground. You need your legs to be comfortable holding up your body. Exercising the legs regularly can keep them in good enough shape to get you where you need and lift you up and down when needed.

2. Reduce Injury

Keeping the legs strong will help improve the density of the leg bones. Strong bones can help keep seniors mobile longer while helping to reduce the chance of serious injury. Exercising the legs helps maintain balance for daily movement and tasks and keeps the joints lubricated and loose to reduce pain.

3. Movement

The goal of exercise as a senior is to maintain independence. By exercising the legs regularly, you can ensure that you'll be able to get up and participate in activities today and tomorrow. When you lose the strength and stability of your legs, you lose the ability to walk around safely by yourself. Being able to move around means being active, which equals better heart health, energy, and calorie burning. If for no other reason, you should exercise your legs to maintain the ability to walk or get up out of a chair.

4. Weight Management

Keeping your legs strong can help keep your whole body strong. Exercising the legs regularly ensures that you will be able to move around and be active. Staying active is the key to being happy with life. Exercise your legs to keep your joints healthy and the blood flowing. Healthy legs provide the opportunity for more activity and cardio exercise options. These exercises and activities are a great way to burn calories and maintain your desired weight. Aside from diet, activity is the best way to lose weight.

Disclaimer:

Leg exercises can be complex, and it's essential to do them correctly. The legs are important to your well-being so take every precaution not to injure them. Be sure to warm up and use light weights. Being able to exercise again tomorrow and the next day is more important than lifting heavy weights.

Chapter 7 Cardio and Core

Cardio and core are good exercises to group together. They both help to burn fat and build strength and endurance. After a warm-up, cardio and then core session (or vice versa) would be acceptable. The exercises complement each other as the core is often used during cardio workouts supplementally. Core exercises should not affect your ability to perform a cardio exercise, and cardio should not tire out the core muscles.

Cardio is one of the most important exercises any individual can perform. It keeps you going and provides energy as it strengthens the heart. The heart is responsible for keeping the blood pumping and sending oxygen and nutrients around the body and to the muscles. The exciting part of cardio is the longer, and more often you do it, the easier it and other activities become.

Cardio can either be performed at a long intensity, such as a slow walk, or at a high intensity, such as sprinting. Research has found that more prolonged low-intensity exercise is equivalent to short, intense exercise. The difference is that low-intensity exercise will need to be performed for a longer period, while high-intensity workouts can be concise but exhausting.

A HIIT exercise or high-intensity interval training is a type of workout that uses high intensity for short periods over and over. Between the intense exercise, there is a period of rest. These exercises are great for building cardio fitness, improving explosive power, and burning fat. This would be the opposite of an endurance exercise like an hour's walk. HIIT can be performed with or without equipment and can consist of jumping, cycling, or sprinting as fast as possible for 15-30 second bursts. HIIT is a valuable tool but be sure to get cleared by a physician before participating in high-intensity exercise.

The core is the center of our body that holds it all together. A strong core provides a good foundation for movement and strength. By keeping our core strong, we can help prevent bad posture and keep ourselves sitting and standing upright. You use your core much more than you think, as it's constantly working to keep us supported. The goal of core exercises isn't to necessarily get a sculpted stomach but to build strength so that you can enjoy daily activities.

Disclaimer: be sure to warm up before any cardio exercises. These workouts often involve the whole body and a lot of movement. It is vital to be loose and prepared to move safely while performing cardio exercises.

Home Workout for Legs with No Equipment

Walking

Walking seems like a simple activity, but it is incredibly powerful. By walking, we are using the muscles, joints, and energy system the body needs to keep strong to continue walking. A walk can be fast or slow, and the duration can vary, but it is an activity that should be done as often as possible as it requires no equipment.

1. Wear comfortable clothes and shoes to walk in.
2. Plan a time or distance you wish to walk. This can vary from day to day or week to week, depending on how you're feeling.
3. Plan out an area to walk in.
4. Go for a walk. Walks should be around at least 30 minutes at a time if possible. Building up to 30 minutes a day may be required.
5. Cool down and stretch appropriately after walking.

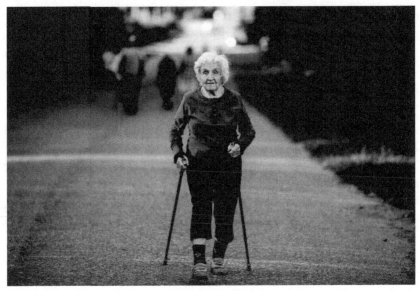

82. A senior on a walk

Dancing

Dancing is an excellent option for cardio. It can be performed inside or outside, and it's a way to keep exercise fun. While you're moving to the music, you are burning calories and strengthening the heart. A dance session can even boost your energy by improving circulation.

1. Find an open area to dance in safely.

2. Wear comfortable clothing and proper footwear for dance movements.

3. Put on your favorite music to move to.

4. Dance along to the music. Try to engage your whole body as you dance.

5. dance sessions should be about 30 minutes if possible. You can take breaks between songs or split the dance sessions into two 15 minutes workouts.

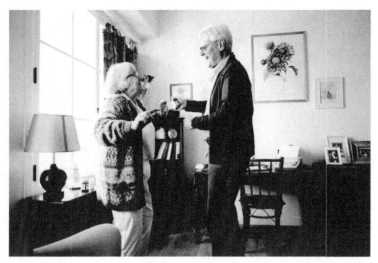
83. Seniors dancing

Planks

Planks are a simple but effective way to strengthen the core. There are many variations, but this is the basic plank and a good starting point for seniors. To make this move more challenging, raise your knees and lower legs, using only your forearms and toes to hold you off the ground.

1. Find an open space where you can lie face down on the floor with your legs extended.

2. Lie face down and prop yourself up on your forearms shoulder-width apart and knees together. Your thumbs should be pointed towards the sky and your palms facing one another. Your lower legs can either lie flat together on the ground or be held together in the air.

3. Exhale. Engage your core and push up through your hips to raise them off the ground. Your thighs and upper body should be up off the ground. Support yourself with your forearms and knees as focal points.

4. Breathe as you hold yourself up for 10-30 seconds.

5. Lower yourself down to the floor. Repeat this movement for three to five sets of 10-30 second holds at a time. Rest for 60 seconds between sets.

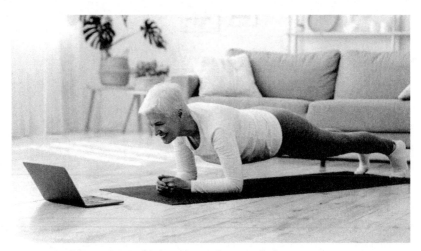

84. A senior performs a plank

Arm and Leg Raise

This is a core strengthening exercise.

1. Find an open space on the floor where you can extend your arms and legs safely.

2. Get down on the floor on your hands and knees. Shoulders should be directly over wrists, and hips should be directly over your knees. Keep the back straight and the neck neutral.

3. Engage the core. Exhale. Lift your left arm straight out in front of you as if reaching for someone.

4. At the same time, lift your right leg straight out behind you. If you cannot lift both at the same time, you can alternate lifting your arm only and then leg only. When the arm and leg are raised, it should form a line with the rest of the body parallel to the floor. Hold the raised position for 5-10 seconds.

5. Inhale as you lower the arm and leg back down. Repeat this for the other arm and leg.

6. Perform this exercise for five sets for each arm and leg combination. Rest 30-60 seconds between sets.

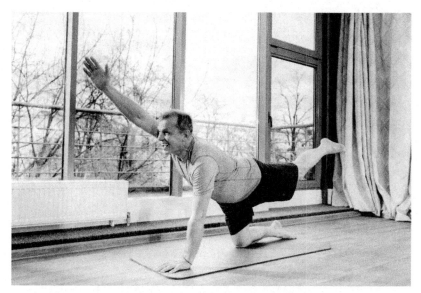
85. A man performs the arm and leg raise.

Bridge

The floor bridge is a safe and effective movement for building core and leg strength. Be sure to engage the core while performing this movement, especially on *core days.*

1. Lie on the ground face up. Bend your knees so your feet are planted flat on the ground about hip-width apart. Extend your arms and place your hand palms down on the ground beside your body.

2. Keep a neutral neck. Engage your core and exhale. Push through your feet and squeeze your buttocks (also known as glutes) to raise your buttocks and lower back up off the floor. Press up through your hips. Your thighs and body will form a straight line, and your knees will be at a 90-degree angle at the top of this movement. The top of your back, shoulders, feet, and head will remain on the ground.

3. Inhale as you lower back down into the starting position. Your back and buttocks should be on the floor and your knees back to a smaller angle.

4. Repeat this movement for three sets of 10-12 reps. Rest for 30-60 seconds between sets.

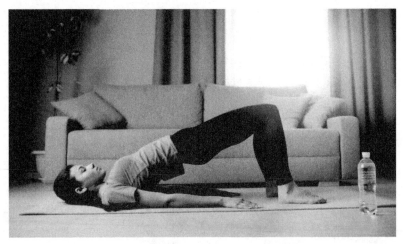
86. A young lady performing a floor bridge.

Home Cardio and Core Workout with Equipment

These exercises will require some equipment to perform. These items will either be found at a sports store, big-box store, or online.

Weighted Walk

1. Get a pair of small dumbbells about 2 lb. or less. Wear comfortable clothes and walking shoes. Plan a distance or time to walk. 30 minutes a day is the recommended minimum for daily cardio activity. Since there is added difficulty due to the weights, performing this walk for a shorter period of time might be best – until fitness is built up.

2. Plan a safe area to walk your scheduled distance or time.

3. Take the dumbbells with you as you walk, and they will add additional resistance and calorie burn. The additional effort from moving with the weight will improve cardio fitness and build arm, grip, and core strength.

4. Be sure to cool down and stretch after your walk.

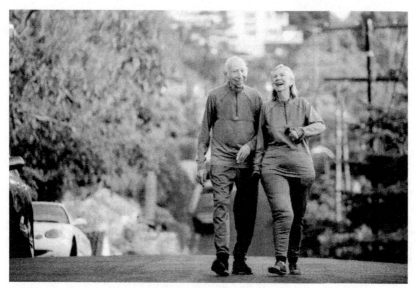
87. A senior walking with weights.

Farmer's walk

This exercise will require a set of dumbbells or other weighted objects from around the house. Since the distance is shorter, if possible, a heavier set of weights should be used than when going for weighted walks.

1. Get a pair of dumbbells or heavy objects.

2. Find a space inside or outdoors in which you can walk back and forth. The strip should be at least 8 large strides long.

3. Lift the dumbbells with one in each hand so they are resting by your pockets.

4. Exhale and step forward. Breathe as you confidently walk for about 8 paces while keeping the weights controlled by your sides. Don't allow the weights to swing or bounce off your thighs

5. After 8 steps or at the end of your space, carefully turn around. Pause briefly to get set and exhale before stepping confidently back down the line for another 8 paces.

6. Walk back and forth three times. Rest for 30 seconds between sets.

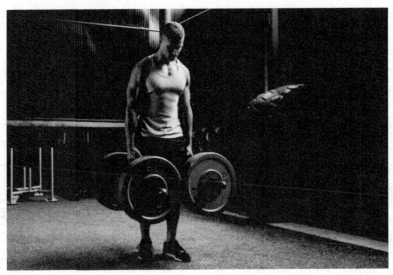
88. A man performs a heavy farmer's walk

Hand Bike

1. A hand bike is a piece of equipment that allows you to do cardio without using your legs. It requires you to pedal using your arms on a surface like a table. You will likely have to order a hand bike online. It is a great alternative to cardio that involves your legs.

1. Get a sturdy table and chair. The table must have enough space for the hand bike to fit comfortably on it. You will need a clock, stopwatch, or another item to time your workout duration.

2. Sit in the chair and move it so you can adequately rotate the pedals of the bike without having to move or stretch.

3. Keep your back straight and head up with a neutral neck.

4. Place your hands on the pedals of the hand bike.

5. Carefully rotate the pedals by moving your arms around in a circular motion.

6. It is best to slowly build up the time you spend on the hand bike. Eventually, it can be a cardio exercise that lasts 15 minutes or more at a time.

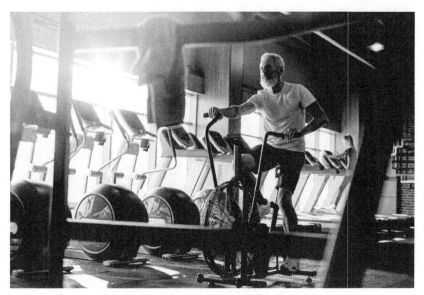
89. A man uses the hand bike.

Seated Straight Leg Lifts

Leg lifts are a core movement that can be performed safely in a sturdy chair.

1. Sit in a sturdy chair placed where you can stretch out your legs in front of it.

2. Scoot forward in the chair and extend your legs. Rest your heels on the ground in front of you. Your legs should form a straight line at about a 45-degree angle from the floor. Support yourself by keeping your hands on the tops of your thighs or holding onto the sides of the chair.

3. Keep a straight back and your chest up. Engage your core. Exhale and slowly raise your right leg up until it is parallel to the ground.

4. Pause briefly at the top before breathing in and lowering your heel back down to the floor. Switch legs.

5. Complete three sets of 8 reps for each leg. Rest for 30-60 seconds between sets.

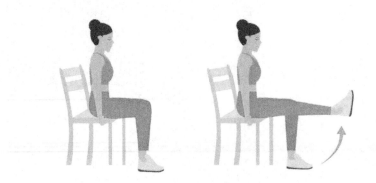

90. A woman performs seated straight leg lifts.

Seated Oblique Stretch

The oblique stretch works the muscles on the sides of the abdomen.

1. Sit tall in a sturdy chair without arms.

2. Place your right hand behind your head with your elbow pointing to your right. Point your left arm straight down by your left side.

3. Engage your core. Inhale and reach down with the left hand towards the floor. Allow your body to lean towards the left side. Your right elbow should point higher towards the sky as your head leans toward the left side.

4. Exhale. Use your core to pull your body from the left and back up to neutral.

5. Switch sides and repeat.

6. Perform two sets of 8-10 repetitions for each side. Rest for 30 seconds between sets.

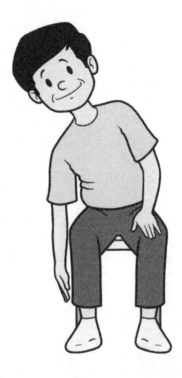

91. A man performs a Seated Oblique Stretch

Gym Workout for Cardio and Core

These workouts should be done using equipment available at the gym.

Elliptical Machine

1. Find an elliptical machine, either seated or standing. The elliptical will have movable arms and legs, and the leg area will have large feet-shaped platforms for your feet. Be sure to warm up properly before cardio exercises.

2. Carefully step onto the feet platforms while grasping the handles for support. Adjust the handles or seat if necessary, so you can adequately extend your arms and legs without stretching on the machine. Many machines will allow you just to start moving on them without having to set anything specific like resistance.

3. Set a time duration and resistance level on the machine if desired. The higher resistance will make it more difficult but will also help improve your back, arm, chest, and leg strength. Grasp the handles and move your arms back and forth while pedaling up and down with your feet on the foot platforms. Keep your back straight and neck neutral while exercising.

4. Continue this movement for 30 minutes, if possible, for low impact on your joints with a high cardio benefit. Be cautious while getting on and off the machine, as it has multiple moving parts.

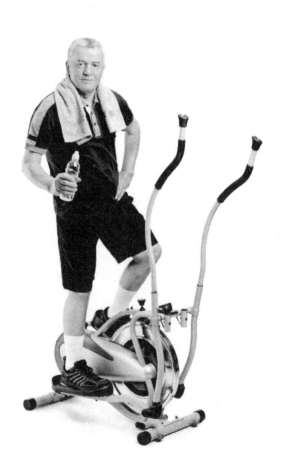

92. A senior on an elliptical machine.

Recumbent Bike

1. Find a recumbent bike at the gym.

2. Adjust the seat so you can adequately extend your legs without stretching too far while pedaling. Adjust the pedal straps so that they securely fit your feet.

3. Adjust the settings on the bike to a specific time, distance, and resistance level. Many bikes will allow you to just pedal without adjusting anything if you choose.

4. Keep your back straight and head up. Push the pedals with your feet and hold on to the handlebars for stability.

5. Continue pedaling at your desired pace for 30 minutes or more if possible.

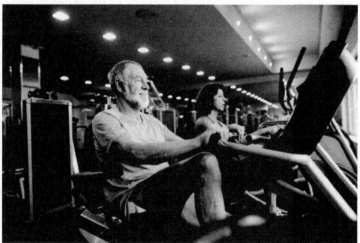

93. Seniors using the recumbent bike.

Treadmill Walk

The treadmill is an excellent cardio option for walking in a safe place, out of the elements, and with the option to add an incline easily.

1. Find the treadmill in the gym. It will be a flat track with arms on the side and a large control panel at the front. Be sure to warm up before cardio exercises.

2. Step onto the stopped treadmill and start the program using the control panel. You will need to adjust the speed and the incline numbers. Start with low speed and no incline to get

started.

3. Once you increase the speed on the machine, the treadmill will start moving. Walk along to the pace of the treadmill. Keep your chest up and neck neutral. Use the support railings on the side if necessary or for getting off the treadmill.

4. To slow down or stop the machine, reduce the speed or hit the emergency stop button. To increase the intensity, add an incline to the walk to walk uphill.

5. Try to walk continuously for at least 30 minutes if possible. You can always stop the treadmill and rest before continuing the workout and completing the 30 minutes.

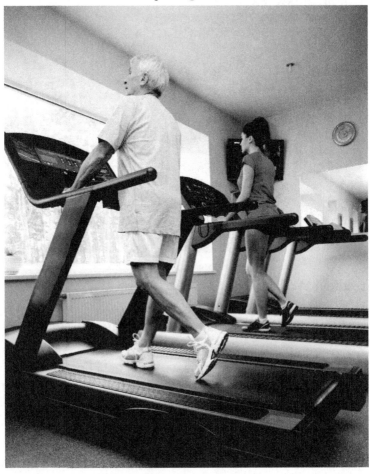

94. A senior walks on a treadmill.

Pallof Press

The Pallof Press uses the cable machine to help improve core strength and stability.

1. Find the cable machine. You'll want the side you can stand in front of that allows the cable to hang free with an adjustable height.

2. Adjust the weight so that it is light enough for you to perform this exercise. Attach the single rectangular handle grip to the cable. Adjust the height of the cable to mid-way down the tree.

3. Stand with your right side facing the cable tree. Grasp the handle with both hands, interlocking fingers. Take a sidestep away from the tree. Spread your feet to shoulder-width apart. Twist your body to the right and back to the center to pull the cable tight.

4. The handle should be at chest level and close to the body. The cable will pull you towards the machine, but your abdominals resist the pull.

5. Exhale. Extend your arms in front of your chest, pushing the handle away from your body. Pause for 5 seconds with arms fully extended, holding the handle.

6. Inhale and slowly bring the handle back in front of your chest.

7. Repeat the movement for three sets of 10 reps. Hold for 5-10 seconds each time you extend your arms. Rest for 30-60 seconds between sets. Switch sides and repeat the sets and reps on the left side.

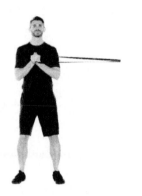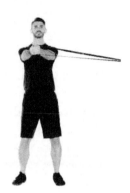

95. A man performs the Pallof Press.

Exercise Ball Leg Balances

An exercise ball is a versatile tool for spicing up exercises and performing core movements. The exercise ball is a giant inflatable ball that most gyms should have.

1. Find an exercise ball, a yoga mat, and an open space inside the gym. If you need to, you can use a smaller exercise ball as it will be slightly easier. You can also start this exercise with no ball to begin.

2. Lie down on the mat facing up. Hold the exercise ball in your hands over your chest. Keep your legs hip-width apart with the knees bent about 90 degrees.

3. Raise your legs up off the ground. Your knees should be directly over your hips, and your lower legs should be parallel to the ground.

4. Place the exercise ball on top of your shins. Balance the ball there. Keep your arms extended, palms on the floor by your sides for support.

5. Engage your core. Inhale and slowly extend your legs out with the ball balanced.

6. Exhale and carefully pull your legs back until they are in the starting position.

7. Repeat this movement while keeping the ball balanced for three sets of 5-8 reps. Rest for 60 seconds between sets.

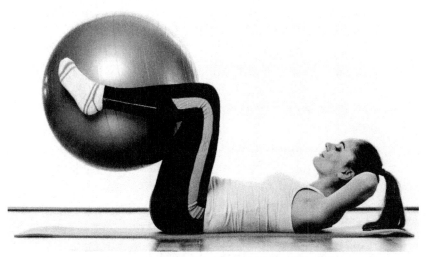

96. A woman balances and exercise ball on her legs.

Partner Workout for Cardio and Core

These exercises are meant to be done with a partner for safety and support. Partners should provide motivation while ensuring their training partner gets through the workout safely.

Suitcase Carry Relay

You will need one or two dumbbells, kettlebells, or another weighted object like a purse for this exercise. The suitcase carry combines core and cardio as you walk while keeping the core engaged.

1. Grab a dumbbell and find a straight open space where you can take 8-10 paces in a row. This exercise may benefit from a heavier weight as you will only be carrying one.

2. Partner 1 will lift the dumbbell in their right hand, and it should rest hanging in the area of their pants' right pocket. Partner 2 will stand beside partner 1, facing the same direction.

3. Engage your core and walk confidently across the space while carrying the weight by your side. Do not swing the weight or allow it to move. Keep a straight back and neutral neck. Try not to lean over in the direction of the weight. Use your core to maintain proper posture and walk as normally as possible.

4. Partner 1 should walk to the other side of the space, carefully turn around, and walk back to the left side of partner 2 and hand off the weight to partner 2's left hand. Partner 2 should then walk across the space just as partner 1 did.

5. Partner 2 should engage the core and walk back across the space confidently. Keep a straight back and use your core to maintain proper walking posture.

6. On this return, Partner 2 should pass the weight to Partner 1's left side. The weight can be handed off or placed on the floor for Partner 1 to pick up.

7. Partner 1 will perform the same routine carrying the weight in the left hand.

8. Though alternating, partners should each walk out and back twice total while holding the weight in the right hand and then out and back twice total while holding the weight in the left hand.

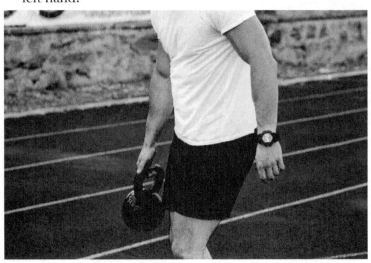

97. A man performs a suitcase carry.

Walk and Talk

1. Plan a meeting with your partner somewhere you can walk for some distance together.

2. Agree on the duration or the distance that you both can walk.

3. Meet up and walk together. Talking during the walk makes the time fly and helps improve your cardio.

4. At least 30 minutes of daily cardio is recommended if possible.

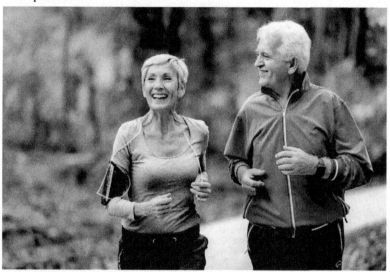

98. Seniors walking together.

Ball Toss

This exercise can be completed using an exercise ball, standard basketball, or soccer ball. The ball toss combines cardio, balance, and abdominal strength.

1. Grab an exercise ball and find an open area where partners can stand a short distance from each other.

2. Partners should spread out and face one another. Keep your legs shoulder-width apart and your back straight.

3. Partner 1, lift the ball in front of your body to about chest height. Engage the core. Exhale and throw the ball towards partner 2 by bouncing it one time off the ground in between you.

4. Partner 2, catch the ball. Set your feet again if you had to move. Engage the core. Exhale and bounce the ball back to partner 1.

5. Partners can throw the ball slightly to the side of one another to encourage more movement when catching it.

6. Throw the ball back and forth for 15 minutes while chatting.

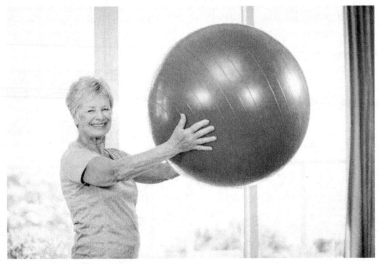

99. A senior holding an exercise ball.

Back-to-Back Ball Pass

For this exercise, you will need an exercise ball, basketball, or another similar ball. A heavier ball can be used if both partners have adequate fitness levels.

1. Partners should either stand or sit back-to-back based on fitness level.

2. Keep legs hip-width apart. If sitting, keep knees bent and feet planted on the floor. If standing, keep knees slightly bent.

3. Partner 1 will begin by holding the ball at the midpoint of the body. Bend elbows to about 90 degrees and keep arms shoulder length apart.

4. Partner 1 will engage the core, exhale, and carefully twist to the left while holding the ball.

5. Partner 2 will twist to the left simultaneously to receive the ball. Partner 1 will release the ball, and partner 2 will grab it.

Partners 1 and 2 will inhale and return to the center.

6. Partner 2 will twist to the left while holding the ball at the midpoint of the body with elbows bent. Partner 1 will twist right to receive the ball.

7. Continue passing the ball around the bodies. Partners should twist 10 times to their right and 10 times to their left for a single set. Rest for 60 seconds between sets. Partners should each perform two to three sets total.

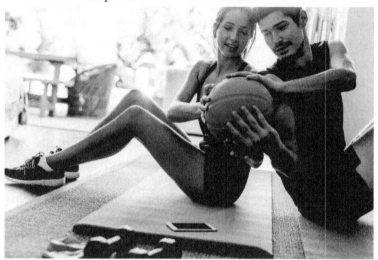

100. Adults performing a back-to-back ball pass.

Cardio and Core Workout Benefits

Cardio and core work together because they keep you supported and moving daily. You use cardio and core fitness more frequently than you realize. You would notice very quickly if your cardio was poor or your core was too weak, and life would become more difficult. There are many benefits to exercising the core and performing cardio.

Benefits:

1. Endurance

Cardio is what keeps you going throughout the day. By training cardio, you are building up your ability to keep going. The more cardio exercise you do, the longer you can be active and full of life. Cardio strength is the strength to walk up the stairs instead of having to stop and catch your breath.

2. Reduce Injury

Cardio keeps your heart pumping. Without cardio, the heart would begin to weaken. Cardio helps to reduce your chances of heart disease and other help conditions. By performing cardio, you are taking an extra "pill" that the doctor can't give you to protect your overall health. Cardio can help boost the immune system and keep the joints fresh. Cardio is an overall protective form of exercise that the body requires. A strong core can help keep us from falling over when you bend or reach for an object. A strong core helps support a strong back and upper body. The core is also crucial for movements like squatting down and standing back up without wobbling or toppling over.

3. Movement

Cardio allows you to move. If you build up cardio, you can move a lot. The more cardio you do, the more energy you will have to stay awake when you want to play with your grandkids or pets. Cardio is activity, and activity is one of the top essentials required for a happy and healthy life. Training your core allows you to move more fluidly and freely. The core supports your body and helps you perform most of the daily tasks you complete without even noticing. By keeping the core strong, you can keep going longer and maintain stability as you age.

4. Weight Management

Cardio is the answer to how to lose weight. By maintaining cardio, you keep up with the calories you need to burn. Cardio is the best way to beat the unwanted body fat or help you drop a few pounds for your health. Cardio helps keep you going and the joints loose, so you can continue to stay active and manage your weight daily.

Disclaimer:

Cardio is an essential part of fitness, but it is crucial to speak to your physician to ensure you are healthy enough for certain exercises. Cardio can be challenging, and there are risks of falling or being out far from home on a walk, for example. Speak to your doctor and call your partner if you have any concerns about your safety when performing these exercises.

Chapter 8 Essential Equipment

Exercise can and should be enjoyable. It does take effort, but eventually, it should feel good. Exercise is like small games that help power up your body through activities. The many equipment options are one aspect of exercise that can be both negative and positive. Equipment can be a motivator for those who don't want to waste their investment but can also turn some users off who aren't sure what and what not to buy.

Exercise generally requires some equipment. The more equipment you have, the more options you have for exercise selection. This can benefit some who get bored quickly by the same exercise or those who have more advanced goals they are trying to reach by diversifying. Equipment isn't necessary, though, to get a good workout in. You can quickly just start moving, such as in the case of dancing for cardio.

The equipment aspect of exercise can be overwhelming because every level has many choices. Now that you have all the exercises to maintain your fitness, we will review the equipment you may or may not need to perform those exercises. We will also provide some insight into how necessary the various equipment is to fitness. Selecting and buying equipment can be a positive motivator for exercise as it will serve as a reminder to work out and as a fun and personalized aspect of the whole process.

Here are some options regarding equipment and guidance on what these items can help with.

Dumbbells

Essential.

Dumbbells are a significant part of fitness and are used in nearly every weight training program. Dumbbell training can help build strength, lose weight or maintain the ability to perform functional movements.

Dumbbells come in many shapes and weights. It's best to start low when first starting with an exercise program, and it's also recommended to get a few different weights if possible. Having dumbbells provides the option for exercise at home. They are the foundation of many of the exercises you should be performing.

Positives

- Dumbbells don't take up too much space as they can be stacked against a wall or hidden under a bed.

- They're easy to use as you can grab one and start moving it around to perform many exercises.

- They provide different exercise options and variations when one is used instead of a set.

Negatives

- They are somewhat expensive. They usually cost somewhere around the same amount as the actual listed weight. While they can be expensive, they last a long time and can be used daily.

They can be dangerous because they are heavy and unforgiving. You can drop a dumbbell or kick a dumbbell on the floor and possibly hurt yourself. Dropping a resistance band won't do as much damage, but they have their own set of drawbacks.

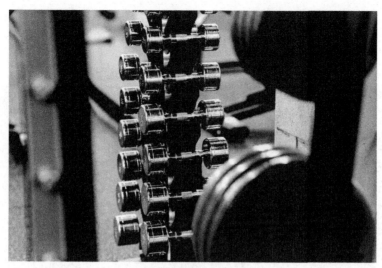
101. A dumbbell rack.

Barbells

Not essential.

Barbells work very similarly to dumbbells. They have a long, weighted bar that requires weight plates to be loaded onto them for exercise. They are used to build strength, are a major part of fitness, and are used in most weight training programs.

Barbells can be a great option for weightlifters, bodybuilders, and those who have adequate space at home where they work out. With a barbell, you can perform compound and full-body movements such as squats and deadlifts.

Positives

- Great for big movements
- You can load a lot of weight onto a barbell for heavier lifting
- They last a long time. Barbells and their weights are very durable

Negatives

- They take up space. The bar is long and usually heavy, and the plates are usually larger than kitchen plates.
- The plates will have to be purchased separately. The plates on a barbell will have to be purchased in sets since both sides of the bar are loaded. This means possibly buying many plates to get a full workout in.

- You need space to perform the movements with a barbell. While the barbell is a great tool, you will need an open space and possibly a large and expensive squat rack to help perform some exercises with it.

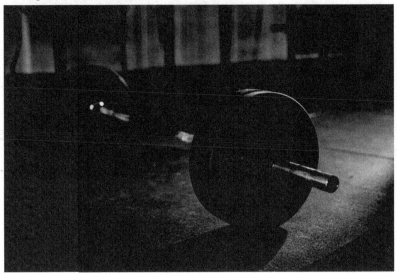

102. A barbell loaded with weight plates.

Resistance bands

Not essential, but recommended.

Resistance bands are a great alternative to dumbbells. They are lightweight and take up no space but can provide resistance for strength training. Resistance bands can also help with certain rotational or pull movements that are superior to dumbbells. Resistance bands come in many different weights and types; there are handled and unhandled versions.

One of the more important roles of resistance bands is providing therapy. They can be used for stretching maneuvers and exercise for those that can't use weights because of physical restrictions. While they are a great tool, they aren't necessary for a good workout.

Positives

- Resistance bands are often prescribed to seniors as a safer option than actual weights. They may put less strain on the joints.

- They are small and lightweight, so you aren't at risk of dropping them and causing injury. You can quickly drop a resistance band with little consequence if it's too much for you.

- Resistance bands are easy to store or bring with you as they can be shoved in a small bag or drawer.

Negatives

- They can snap back and hurt you if you are not careful. While it's not incredibly common, a resistance band could come unfastened or break and snap back at the user.

- You may need something to attach them to while performing many exercise movements. While you can pick up a dumbbell and start lifting, resistance bands often require a setup with an anchor to hold the other end of the band.

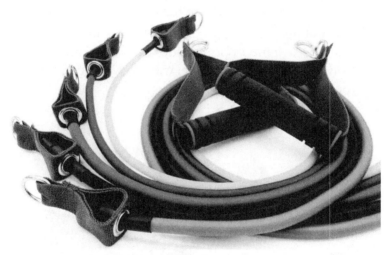

103. A resistance band set with handles.

Jump Rope

Not essential.

The jump rope is a piece of traditional exercise equipment that's great for cardio. Jumping rope is a straightforward exercise, but it's not for everyone. It's not the best idea for seniors to jump around as many have physical restrictions, plus their aging joints won't appreciate the strain.

Jumping rope is a recommended exercise for many, but it's not the best choice for seniors. It requires rhythm and speed to perform the movement and consistent hopping.

Positive

- Jump ropes are inexpensive and can be purchased in many places for a good price.

- Jump ropes can be stored conveniently as they roll or fold up to a compact size.

- Jumping rope is a cardio exercise that can be done alone at home with great results.

Negative

- Jumping rope requires a lot of movement, which isn't safe for many seniors.

- Jumping rope can be dangerous even for experienced exercisers. Jump ropes can easily trip you or whip you in the face while trying to perform the movement.

- You will need a decent amount of space to jump rope. You can take a jump rope outside, but many like to exercise indoors, and jumping rope will likely require rearranging your workout space.

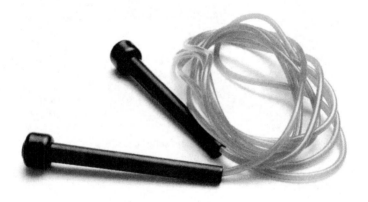

104. A rolled-up jump rope.

Running Shoes/Walking Shoes

Essential.

Good running shoes are an essential piece of exercise equipment; they provide a measure of safety while boosting performance during exercise. Finding the right shoe for running or walking can make the required movement feel better and reduce the strain it puts on the joints. Sports-specific shoes can be used for running, walking, strength exercises, and even yoga.

Shoes can also be a great motivator. Shopping for and finding the right shoes can keep an exerciser motivated to try out and continue to use their new purchase. Running and walking shoes come in a large variety. The options may be overwhelming for some but are beneficial because they provide for different feet, steps, and styles that benefit the wearer.

Positive

- Shoes can help motivate you to get up and use them for exercise.
- They can help reduce joint pressure or pain when walking and running
- They last for a long time and can be used for a functional activity like going for a walk at the store.

Negative

- There are many kinds of shoes to choose from, which can be overwhelming.
- Walking and running shoes can be expensive. While there are cheaper options, some of the better-quality shoes will cost you more than a beginning may want to spend
- Finding the correct shoe takes time and effort, which may be discouraging. It can also cause the wearer trouble if the wrong shoe is selected.

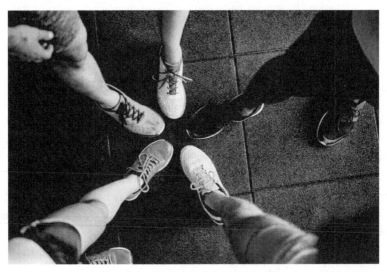
105. Adults displaying their running shoes.

Ab Wheel

Not essential.

The ab wheel is a specific piece of exercise equipment that targets the core by having the user roll out their upper body on their knees using extended arms. The movement is challenging, but the results can be clearly felt. The ab wheel is a smaller item that is good when it comes to storage, but it takes a little room to use it. The ab well is a strength-building exercise that targets the core.

While the ab wheel is an excellent piece of equipment for core exercises, it's not essential. The ab wheel takes a lot of strength and skill and is likely unsuitable for many seniors. It can put a strain on the shoulder and lower back. The ab wheel is likely for more advanced exercisers or bodybuilders. A plank is a much safer option that can be done anywhere without equipment.

Positives

- Very effective at strengthening the core
- It only takes up a little storage space
- It can be used in a small space like the living room

Negative

- Not a functional movement that works toward your goal of maintaining independence

- Puts strain on the joints that can be discouraging or sideline an exerciser
- It takes a good deal of strength to use and is more suited to those with an established level of fitness

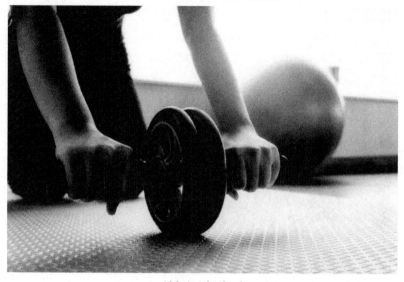

106. An ab wheel

Yoga Mat

Necessary.

A yoga mat is a thin mat that can be rolled out to provide an exercise surface. The mat is used during yoga classes to define the space in which the exerciser should stay, giving them a clean and safe place to perform their movements. It can serve as your exercise space and even be a motivator as its style and color can be personally selected. Yoga mats are soft and made of a texture that provides extra grip.

While a yoga mat isn't used for any movement, it is where your movements will be performed. It will give you a safe place with an additional grip to stand and perform your movements. Yoga mats can be used as your spot for strength movements, in-place cardio, stretching, or yoga.

Positives

- Yoga mats are relatively cheap and easy to find

- They are simple to put away and store somewhere out of the way
- They help prevent rug burns or injury from slipping on a surface like a wood floor

Negatives

- They aren't necessary to perform for any workout but make many workouts easier and safer
- They do take up space when rolled out that some may not have in their household

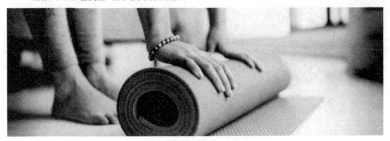

107. A partially rolled yoga mat.

Fitness Clothing

Essential.

The clothing you exercise in matters. While you can still perform movements in your regular clothes, it doesn't always feel good and isn't always safe. Fitness clothing provides a lightweight option that allows you to move freely. Fitness clothes are very functional and can be used for cardio, strength training, or even yoga.

The clothes you select for your workout could either motivate or discourage you. Fitness clothing provides the exerciser with something they can personally select to feel comfortable and confident when exercising. Exercise clothes also protect the exerciser's everyday clothes from getting damaged during a workout

Positives

- Selecting and wearing fitness clothes can be a source of motivation
- Provides restriction-free movement
- Protects the exerciser's other clothing from damage while working out

Negatives

- There are so many choices that they can become discouraging to some
- Some brands and styles of fitness clothing can get expensive
- It's not necessary to perform any workout but is much more practical than regular clothing

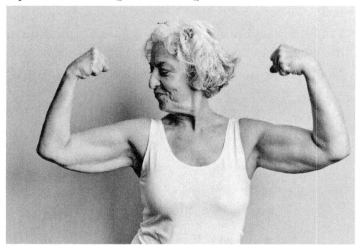

108. An older adult proudly wearing a fitness top.

Exercise Ball

Not essential but recommended for seniors.

The exercise ball is a large rubber inflatable ball used for various exercises. The exercise ball doesn't weigh much, but it is awkwardly large and can bounce. It is used for strength, cardio, stability, and balance exercises. While using an exercise ball is not necessary, it can be very beneficial to seniors trying to maintain stability and balance.

Exercise balls provide a fun tool to spice up some workouts while making others possible at home. These can be found at most stores and often come with their own way to inflate the ball. There can be some difficulty getting used to using an exercise ball, and the exercises can also prove challenging to some users.

Positives

- Build stability and balance
- A fun addition to incorporate into any workout

- Increases the number of exercises that can be performed
- Doesn't weigh too much, and dropping it isn't very dangerous

Negatives

- An inflated exercise ball is large and takes up a lot of space. There isn't really any good place to store an inflated exercise ball.
- Could pop and result in the user falling a short distance to the ground unexpectedly
- Not necessary to maintain your fitness or exercise in general

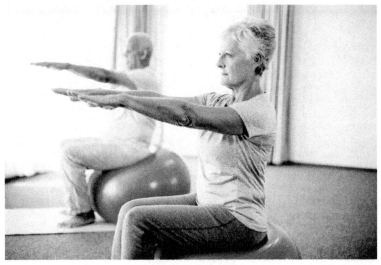

109. Seniors using exercise balls.

Step Platform

Essential.

The step platform adds another level to many workouts. It is simply a small rectangular step that can be placed on flat ground for the user to step onto. The platform provides a lot of functional exercise options for exercisers to perform. Although it is simply a single step, it adds a new dimension and degree of difficulty to many workouts. Step platforms can build strength, improve balance and stability, and even be used for cardio movements.

The step platform does take up space as it's a rectangular board large enough to stand on safely. Those with their own step in their house likely will not be interested in a platform. However, it's an excellent tool for seniors or those trying to maintain the ability to perform functional movements.

Positives

- Adds many exercise movements to your arsenal
- Although it requires a step up, the platform is relatively safe and likely safer than a household step option

Negatives

- The step platform will take up space to store
- To perform some movements on the step platform, you'll need a decent amount of space
- They can be expensive, especially for a beginner to invest in

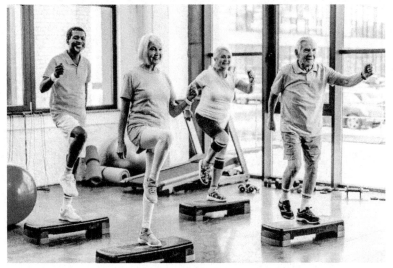

110. Seniors using a step platform

Wrist Wraps

Not essential.

Wrist wraps are usually made of durable cloth or similar material. They are used for gripping the weights you are lifting or supporting your wrists during a movement. They are used by many heavy lifters and bodybuilders and can be a valuable tool. Wraps are a small and convenient way to improve your lift capacity and add some safety to an otherwise dangerous movement.

Wrist wraps aren't necessary to exercise. They are a personal choice item that may or may not benefit the user. Seniors are not typically lifting heavy or performing very dangerous weight maneuvers, so wrist wraps don't serve them much purpose. They motivate some exercisers as they are fitness-specific pieces of equipment, but for many, they have no use.

Positives

- Wrist wraps are small and easy to store
- They can improve your lift capacity
- They are usually cheap and easy to purchase

Negatives

- They aren't necessary for any movement
- Misusing them could lead to injury
- You may put them away in a sock drawer and lose track of one or both

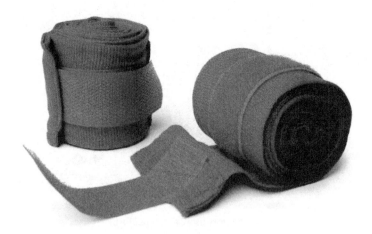

111. A pair of wrist wraps

Chapter 9 Work on Your Joint Strength

While the muscles power you through activity and exercise, the joints keep you together. No matter how strong you are, you're not going anywhere without your joints functioning correctly. The joints help connect the body and keep it a complete well-oiled machine with many working parts. The joints are undoubtedly important, but they age just like the rest of the body and sometimes even faster.

The joints wear down as you age due to time and constant use, and they become frail, stiff, or lose the cushiony cartilage that supports us. All seniors need to pay attention to joint health whether they exercise or not. Keeping joints in good health to keep yourself moving takes some extra time and attention. This extra effort through stretching, diet, and therapeutic exercises can make the difference between being an active or inactive senior.

The joints that cause the most problems include the knees, hips, shoulders, and wrists. By being cognizant of this fact and acting, you can avoid serious issues. We'll go over some diet tips, stretches, and workouts that can serve as a magic pill to help maintain your joints.

Diet

The joints are made up of ligaments, cartilage, bones, and the thick lubricating fluid called synovial fluid. The joints are complex, and they allow us to perform incredible movements. What you eat can directly impact your joints and your ability to move.

The pain and stiffness in most joints are caused by inflammation, which can be caused by diet, overuse, injury, or age. While you can't turn back the clock, you can put the proper nutrients into your body to trick it into feeling younger. An anti-inflammatory diet can help reduce joint pain and increase mobility. Foods that cause inflammation include fried food, processed food, and foods high in sugar.

Anti-inflammatory foods to add to your diet include:

- Nuts
- Milk
- Fish
- Broccoli
- Cauliflower
- Olive Oil
- Beans
- Garlic
- Dark chocolate

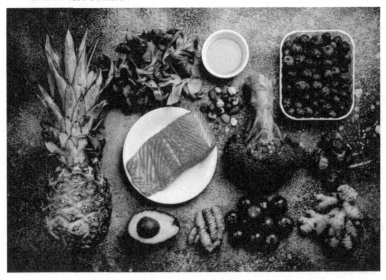

112. A selection of anti-inflammatory foods.

Supplements

There are also supplements available that can help aging joints. Supplements are additions to the diet, usually in pill form, that can provide the body with additional needed nutrients. These supplements can all be purchased at the local drug store, vitamin shop, or in many big-box stores. While your doctor prescribes an anti-inflammatory like ibuprofen for your joints, you can also discuss taking these natural supplements for increased results. These supplements will, through their unique methods, help reduce inflammation while strengthening your joints.

Joint Supplements

- Glucosamine
- Chondroitin
- MSM
- Omega-3
- Vitamin D
- Turmeric

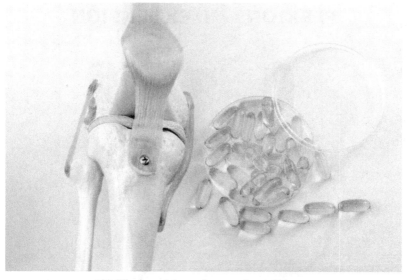

113. The knee joint and omega-3 supplements.

Stretches and Workouts for Joints

Knees

Knee Flexion

For this exercise, you should begin with a chair or counter in front of you for support. You can advance to know support after balance is established.

1. Stand in front of the counter and hold on to it for balance.

2. Feet should be close together. Exhale. Raise the right foot and put it behind you by bending the knee to 90 degrees if possible.

3. Inhale. Lower the foot back down to the ground by straightening the knee.

4. Repeat this for three sets of 10 reps for each leg. Rest for 30 seconds between the sets.

FLEXION AND EXTENSION

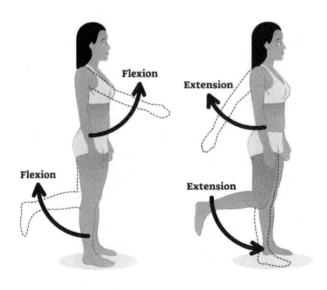

114. A woman demonstrates knee flexion and knee extension

Knee Extensions

1. Sit on a chair or couch high enough so the knees can sit at a 90-degree angle with feet planted on the floor directly below the knees. Move around in the chair if necessary to achieve a position where the chair supports the thighs.

2. Sit up straight in the chair with your chest up and shoulders back. Maintain a neutral neck. Place hands over thighs for support. Exhale. Extend left leg at the knee. Raise the lower part of the leg until it forms a straight line with the rest of the leg parallel to the floor.

3. Inhale and slowly lower the leg back down to the 90- degree angle, starting position.

4. Repeat this movement for three sets of 10 repetitions for each leg. Rest for 30-60 seconds between sets.

Side Steps

1. Stand with feet hip-width apart

2. Step to the left with your left so that your feet are far apart.

3. Take a step close to your left leg with your right leg.

4. Repeat the movement back to the other side

5. Repeat this series 10 times for two to three sets. Rest 30 seconds between sets.

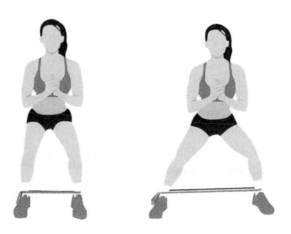

115. A woman demonstrates a side step with a resistance band

Step-Ups

For this exercise, you will need a step platform or another safe flat surface to step up on. A porch step could be used if it is in a safe spot and is not too high.

Note: This exercise can be done from multiple angles to help improve balance on strength when moving or stepping in various directions. You can step on and back off, on and over, laterally(sidestep) on and off, or laterally up and over. You can also begin on the step and step down and back up. Use these different angles to make the workout more challenging or to keep the workout exciting.

1. Stand in front of the step. Your feet should only be slightly apart. Pay attention to where the step is in front of you.

2. Exhale and lead with the right foot; step up onto the step.

3. Follow through by bringing the left foot up onto the step. The step should be a fluid 1-2 movement.

4. Inhale and step off the step leading with your right foot. Follow through with the left.

5. Repeat this movement for three sets of 10-12 reps. Switch legs and lead with the left foot first for another three sets. Rest for 60 seconds between sets.

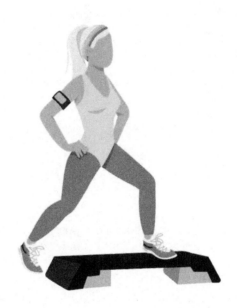

116. A woman steps up onto a step platform

Calf Raises

Depending on your fitness level, for this exercise, you will need a chair for support, no equipment, or a set of light dumbbells. You can begin by using the chair and progress to the dumbbells.

1. Stand with light dumbbells in your hands by your sides. Keep feet close together.

2. Exhale and push up through the balls of your feet. Use your calves to raise your mid feet and heels off the ground. Move slowly and do not bounce.

3. Breathe out and slowly lower yourself down. Once your feet are flat on the ground, lean slightly back on your heels to raise your toes and balls of your feet off the ground.

4. Return to flat foot briefly before repeating the movement from the beginning.

5. Repeat for two sets of 10 repetitions. Rest for 30-60 seconds between sets.

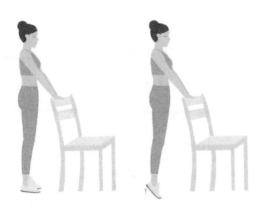

117. A woman demonstrates a supported calf raise

Hips

Standing Hip Flexor

For this exercise, you can hold onto a counter or chair for support until adequate balance is achieved.

1. Stand with your hands on your hips. Take a large step forward with your right foot so your thigh is at a 45-degree angle.

2. Raise your heel up off the left leg and bend your knee.

3. Push your pelvis or hips forward by squeezing your glutes.

4. Hold this position for 30 seconds and then switch legs.

5. Repeat this stretch 2-3 times for each leg.

HIP FLEXOR STRETCH

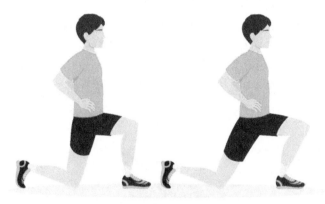

118. A man demonstrates the standing hip flexor stretch

Knee to Chest

1. Lay down and pull your knees up to your chest.
2. Wrap your arms around your bent knees to keep them in place
3. Pull your knees toward your chest and tuck your chin into your chest.
4. Hold this position for 15 seconds
5. Relax by extending legs back out but keeping them raised off the ground.
6. Repeat the stretch for three sets.

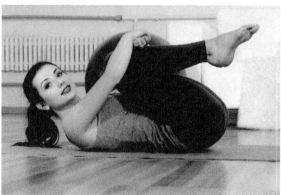

119. A woman performs a knee-to-chest hold

Hip Circles

1. Stand with feet slightly wider than shoulders. Put your hands on your hips and bend your knees.

2. Make big clockwise circles by slowly rotating your hips. Keep your keep and lower legs in place.

3. Rotate around for 30 seconds before switching direction and rotating counterclockwise for 30 seconds.

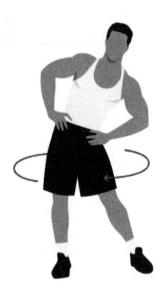

120. A man performing hip circles

Prone Straight Leg Raise

1. Lay face down on the ground.

2. Engage your core and squeeze your buttocks.

3. Exhale. Lift one leg up slowly off the ground keeping the rest of the body down.

4. Hold for 3 seconds at the top before breathing in and lowering the leg.

5. Repeat this movement for two sets of 10 reps for each leg.

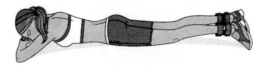

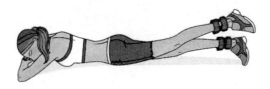

121. A woman performs a prone leg raise.

Hip Abductors

You will need a sturdy chair wall or counter to brace yourself for this exercise.

1. Stand with feet hip-width apart and hold on to the chair in front of you. Keep your back straight and neck neutral.

2. Raise your right leg up to the side and back (diagonally). It's a slight movement. Hold the foot there for 3 seconds.

3. Bring the right foot back in from behind to the starting position.

4. Perform this movement 5 times for each leg.

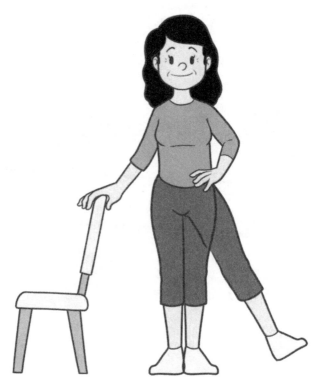

122. A woman performs a standing hip abductor

Shoulders

Shoulder Stretch

1. Sit in a chair. Keep your back straight and chest up.

2. Put your right hand on your left shoulder. Use your left hand to help support your elbow. Try to keep your right elbow at shoulder height.

3. Pull your right elbow toward your left shoulder with your left hand, and you will feel a slight stretch. Once a stretch is felt, hold that spot for 10 seconds.

4. Switch sides. Perform two to three sets for each side.

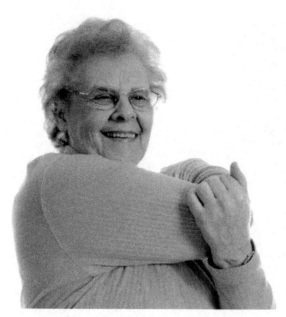

123. A wpman performs a shoulder stretch.

Shoulder Rolls

1. Stand or sit tall with your chest up, neutral spine, and engaged core. Your shoulders should be back and down. Maintain a forward-looking position.

2. Shrug your shoulders as high as you can toward your ears. Do not hunch your back, protrude your neck, or allow your shoulders to slump forward.

3. Squeeze your shoulder blades together and draw your shoulders back once you've shrugged as high as possible.

4. Pull your shoulders down by activating your mid-back.

5. Once you've reached the neutral starting posture, round your upper back slightly to press your shoulders forward while retaining a strong core.

6. Start a new shoulder roll by shrugging up again.

7. Perform three sets of 10 to 15 reps. Rest for 30 seconds between sets.

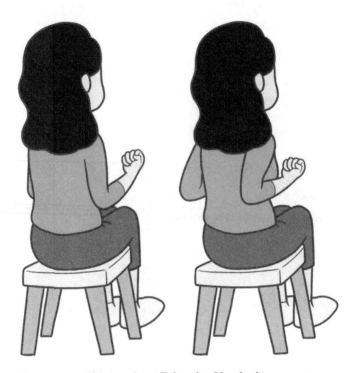

124. A senior rolls her shoulders back.

Shoulder Circles

1. Sit in a chair. Keep your back straight and neck neutral.

2. Reach your hands up and place your fingers on top of your shoulders.

3. While keeping your fingers on your shoulder, circle your shoulders forward.

4. Repeat this movement but circle backward instead.

5. Complete 15 rotations forward and 15 rotations backward. Rest for 30 seconds between directions.

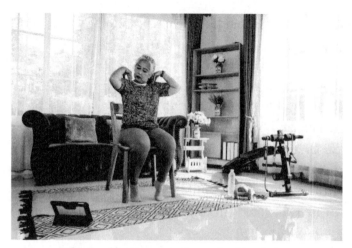

125. An older woman performs shoulder circles.

Overhead Reach

1. Sit in a chair. Keep your back straight and maintain a neutral neck.

2. Interlock your fingers in your lap.

3. Exhale. Raise your arms over your head while keeping your fingers interlocked.

4. Inhale and lower arms back down to your lap.

5. Repeat this movement at least 10 times.

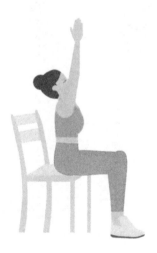

126. A senior performing an overhead reach stretch

Upper Back and Shoulder Stretch

1. Sit in a chair. Keep your back straight, chest up, and maintain a neutral neck.

2. Put your palms together and hold your hands in front of your chest in a prayer position.

3. Exhale and bring your arms overhead.

4. Separate hands and face palms forward.

5. Inhale and squeeze your shoulder blades as you lower your arms out to the sides until they are parallel to the ground.

6. Bring your hands in towards your lap and then up to return to prayer position.

7. Repeat this movement for 15 repetitions.

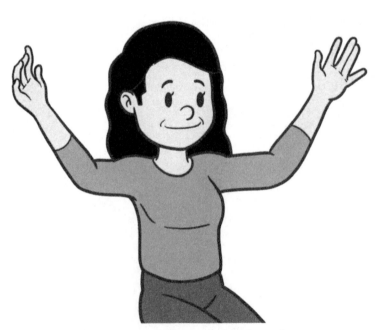

127. A woman performs an upper back stretch.

Wrists

Arm Flexion/Extension

1. Stand or sit in a chair. Keep a straight back and extend your right arm out in front of you.

2. Keep your arm at shoulder height. Use your left arm to support your right arm by grasping it under the forearm.

3. Make a fist with your right hand. Using only your wrist, move your fist up as far as it will go and then slowly down as far as it will go.

4. Continue to put the wrist through its full range of flexion and extension for at least 12 seconds

5. Repeat for the left arm.

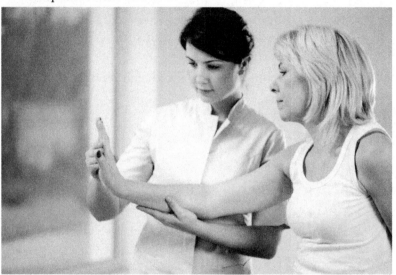

128. A woman stretching her wrist into flexion with assistance.

Thumb Flexion

1. Sit in a chair or stand and keep a straight back and neutral neck. Keep your shoulders down.

2. Hold your hands slightly wider than shoulder length apart, so your palms are facing forward. Hands should be just above shoulder height.

3. Keep your fingers spread wide.

4. Touch your index finger with your thumb and hold for a

second.

5. Open your hand back wide again.

6. Touch your thumb to the middle, ring, and pinky finger in the same fashion.

7. Complete 10 sets of touching every finger once

Wrist Circles

1. Stand tall and hold your arms outstretched in front of you. Maintain balance.

    Modification: If arms can't be held outstretched, elbows can be kept at the sides and bent 90 degrees so that hands are kept straight in front of you. Perform the following steps from this position.

2. Without moving your arms, make outward circles with your wrists as if unwinding a spool of thread. Then repeat the motion making inward circles with your wrist as if winding a thread around a spool.

3. Perform eight outward circles and eight inward circles.

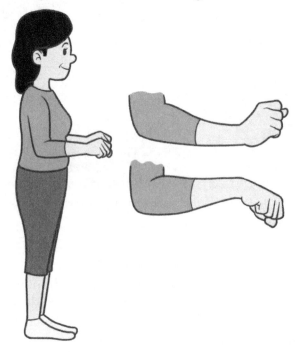

129. A woman performing wrist circles.

Wrist Radial/Ulnar Stretch

1. Stand or sit in a chair. Keep your back straight and your neck neutral.

2. Extend your right arm out in front of you with your thumb pointing towards the ceiling. Try to keep your arm at shoulder height.

3. Make a fist with your right hand. Use your left hand to support your right arm by grasping your right forearm just below the elbow.

4. Using your right wrist, slowly pull your fist down as far as possible.

5. Slowly pull your fist back up and far as possible.

6. Perform five repetitions of up and down for each wrist

Ball Squeeze

For this wrist exercise, you will need a squeezable exercise ball, or you can substitute a rolled-up sock.

1. Sit in a chair or stand. Keep your back straight.

2. Grasp a sock or squeezable ball in your hand.

3. Raise your hand up to above and just in front of your shoulder by bending at the elbow. Keep your palm facing forward.

4. Squeeze the ball with all your fingers and hold for a count of 5.

5. Perform three sets of squeezes for each hand. Rest for 10 seconds between sets.

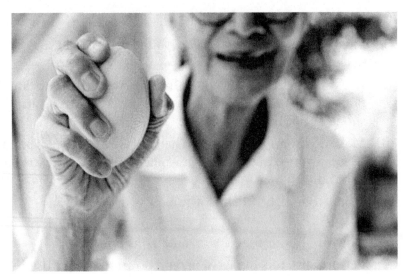
130. A senior performs a ball squeeze.

Disclaimer: While joints commonly tend to be sore as we age, it's not okay to be in pain. If you experience joint pain, it is recommended to speak to your doctor on ways to manage and relieve it. These stretches and exercises can help keep joints healthy but may not be suitable for everyone. Once cleared by your doctor, use these stretches as a personal tool to maintain your independence.

Chapter 10: Building Balance: Yoga and Chair Yoga

While exercise helps maintain the mind, joints, and body, yoga can help uplift them. *Yoga* is an ancient practice that has been around for thousands of years, and it is used to focus the mind and body while focusing on bringing peace to the spirit.

Yoga helps to stretch muscles and loosen the joints while increasing circulation. The movements in yoga will put weight on or stretch the body in different positions that strengthen the muscles and joints. These yoga poses can help build stronger bones, which is essential for seniors.

Seniors can benefit from practicing yoga alongside a well-rounded exercise routine. Yoga incorporates movements that increase flexibility, build strength, and relax the mind. Athletes use yoga regularly to maintain their fitness, flexibility, and focus for their sports. Practicing yoga alongside your exercises can help reduce your chances of injury and muscle recovery time. Improve your balance and build functional strength with yoga

Since yoga uses breathing and stretching together, it reduces stress and can help improve sleep. While seniors may not have full-time jobs anymore, they still have stress, and yoga can help manage it. By reducing stress and promoting better sleep, you can boost your immune system and reduce instances of injury. Yoga day or yoga daily can help you to increase your ability to perform the exercises you need to stay fit while keeping your spirits high.

Yoga Exercises

Cat-Cow

This stretch can be performed in a chair or on the ground, depending on your fitness level and restrictions.

1. Get down onto your hands and knees with palms flat. Keep your shoulders over your wrists and hips directly over your knees. Begin with a straight back.

2. Inhale. Lower your belly, pull your shoulders back, look to the sky and lift your buttocks. This is the "cow" part of the pose.

3. Exhale. Pull your belly in, round your back, tuck your tail bone, put your head down and look toward your belly. This is the "cat" aspect of the pose.

4. Hold each position briefly before switching to the next.

5. Perform three sets of the cat-cow.

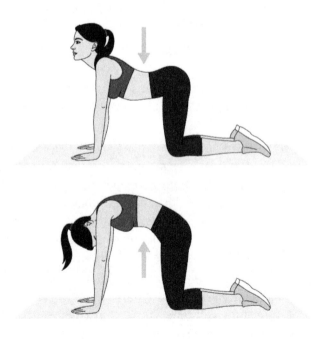

131. A woman demonstrates the cat-cow.

Reverse Arm Hold

This stretch will require a chair.

1. Sit in a chair with your back straight. Move forward so your back is not touching the back of the chair.

2. Inhale and reach your arms out to your sides with a slight bend in the elbow.

3. Keep the arms low as you circle them behind you and grab the opposite wrist behind your lower back

4. Keep your chest and head up. Arch your back slightly as you hold this position for 3 seconds.

5. Return your arms back out to your sides and into your lap in front of you.

6. Perform 3 -5 sets of this movement.

Chair Pigeon

1. You will need a chair for this stretch.

2. Sit in a chair with a straight back. Keep your back off the back of the chair.

3. Carefully pull your left ankle on top of your right knee.

4. Exhale and bend forward at the waist bringing your chest toward your left calf. Hold this position for 5 seconds.

5. Inhale and bring your torso back up to the starting position.

6. Switch sides and repeat.

7. Perform 3 repetitions of this stretch for each leg.

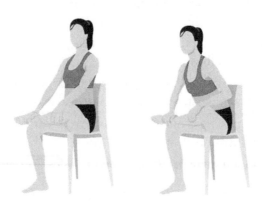

132. A woman demonstrates the chair pigeon pose.

Eagle Arms

You will need a chair for this stretch.

1. Sit in a chair and keep your back straight.

2. Extend your arms out in front of you at about shoulder height. Bend them to 90 degrees at the elbow, so your hands are up over your elbows.

3. Cross your right arm over the left and bring your forearms together. If you can't cross your arms over each other, you can cross your arms and grab the opposite shoulder.

4. Interlock your fingers and raise your elbows. Arch your back slightly.

5. You will feel a stretch in the shoulder and upper back as you raise the elbows up together

6. Hold the stretch for 5 seconds and switch arms.

7. Repeat this 3 times for each arm.

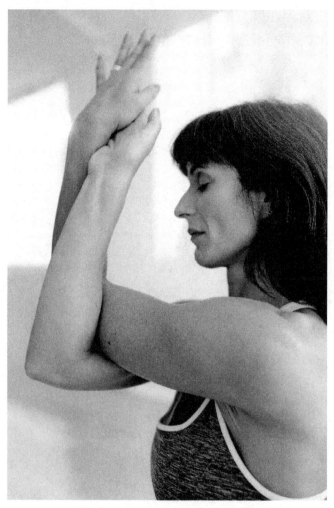

133. A woman demonstrates eagle arms.

Tree Pose

This pose may require a chair or counter for balance.

1. Stand tall in front of a chair. Grab the back of the chair for support.

2. Place your right foot on the left inner thigh or right below the knee.

3. Pull your right leg out to the side while keeping the foot on the opposite thigh.

4. Hold for 8 seconds and switch legs. If you don't need a chair for support, hold your hands in front of your chest in a

prayer position.

5. Perform three sets for each leg.

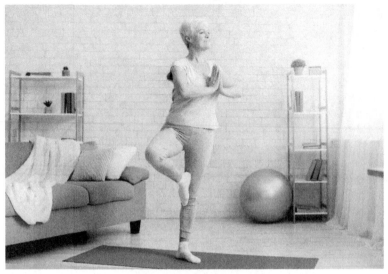

134. A senior practices tree pose.

Sphinx

1. Lie face down on the floor. Put your forearms and palms down on the floor. Your elbows should be below the shoulders.

2. Press down with your arms and pull your shoulder blades back to lift your chest and head up off the floor. Your stomach and legs will remain on the floor.

3. Hold this position for 8 seconds before lowering back down.

4. Repeat this for 5 sets.

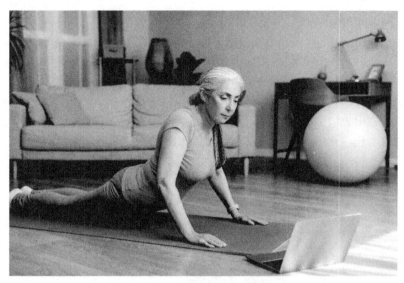

135. Woman performing a sphinx pose.

Cobbler's Pose

1. Sit on the floor and bring the bottoms of your feet together so your knees will open out to the sides.

2. Hold your feet together with your hands.

3. Exhale. Bend forward towards your toes until you feel a stretch. Try not to round the back.

4. Hold for 5 seconds and inhale before slowly coming up.

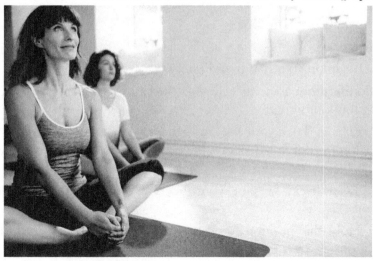

136. A woman seated in a cobbler's pose.

Mountain Pose

1. Stand tall with a straight back and chest up. Keep your feet close together. Open your hands wide by your sides with palms facing forward.

2. Extend up through the spine and gaze up as you keep your head high.

3. Pull your shoulders down and back. Inhale and exhale.

4. Hold for 8 seconds. Repeat this pose 3 times.

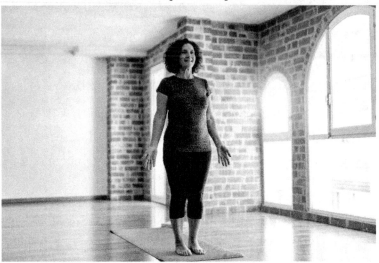

137. A woman performing mountain pose.

Downward Facing Dog

Advanced

1. Begin on your hands and knees.

Modification: You can use your forearms if the pressure is too much for your wrists.

2. Exhale. Tuck your toes, straighten your knees, and raise your hips. Keep your head between your arms and in line with your spine.

3. Lean back, keeping your heels as close to the ground as possible.

4. Hold this position for 8 seconds. Inhale and lower yourself back down to your hands and knees.

5. Perform this hold 3-5 times.

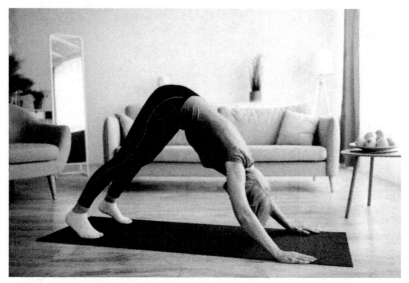
138. An adult performing the downward-facing dog pose.

Warrior 1

Advanced

This exercise can be performed while holding a chair for stability.

1. Stand beside a chair with the chair back near your right hip.
2. Step forward with your right leg but keep your knee over your ankle.
3. Step back with the left leg and turn it slightly outward to a 45-degree angle.
4. Keep your hips centered.
5. Inhale and straighten your right leg to press the body down to feel a stretch. Hold for 3 seconds.
6. Exhale, lift your hips up and bend your right knee back to the original position.
7. Perform three sets of 5 reps for each leg. Move the chair to the otherwise when switching legs.

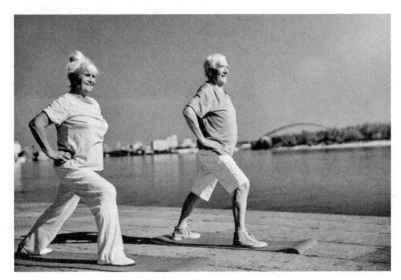
139. Seniors in the warrior 1 pose.

Workout Routines with No Weights

Routine 1: 6 Days Per Week

Week 1

Monday

Back

Warm-ups: Shoulder Rolls, Shoulder Squeezes, Arm Swings

Supermans

Good Mornings

Standing Arm Lifts

Tuesday

Biceps

Warm-ups: Arm Swings Lateral, Arm Swings, Wrist Circles

Biceps Isometric Press

No Weight Curl

Wednesday
Legs

Warm-ups: Leg Swings, Lateral Leg Swings, Standing Knee Bend, Ankle Circles

Chair Squat

Standing Leg Raises

Floor Bridge

Knee Extensions

Thursday
Cardio

Warm-ups: Leg Swings, Shoulder Rolls, Knee Bends, Seated Hamstring Stretch

Go for a walk or dance for 30 minutes

Friday
Core

Warm-ups: Shoulder Rolls, Shoulder Squeezes, Standing Knee Bend

Arm Leg Raise

Plank

Saturday
Yoga

Cat Cow

Eagle Arms

Warrior I

Chair Pigeon

Tree Pose

Sunday

Rest

Week 2

Monday

Chest

Warm-ups: Lateral Arm Swings, Shoulder Squeezes, Neck Stretches

Wall Pushup

Incline Pushup

Pushup

Tuesday

Triceps

Warm-ups: Wrist Circles, Arm Swings, Shoulder Rolls

Dips

Knee Pushups

Wednesday

Shoulders

Warm-up: Shoulder Rolls, Shoulder Squeezes, Neck Stretch, Arm Swings, Lateral Arm Swings

Standing Arm Lifts

Lying Arm Raises

Thursday

Cardio

Warm-ups: Leg Swings, Shoulder Rolls, Knee Bends, Seated Hamstring Stretch

Go for a walk or dance for 30 minutes

Friday

Core

Warm-ups: Shoulder Rolls, Shoulder Squeezes, Standing Knee Bend

Arm Leg Raise

Plank

Saturday

Yoga

Reverse Arm Hold

Mountain Pose

Cobbler's Pose

Downward Facing Dog

Sphinx

Sunday

Rest

Routine 2: Push, Pull, Legs

Week 1

Monday

Push

Warm-ups: Arm Swings, Lateral Arm Swings, Shoulder Rolls

Pushup

Dips

Lying Arm Raise

Plank

Tuesday

Rest

Wednesday

Cardio

Warm-ups: Leg Swings, Shoulder Rolls, Knee Bends, Seated Hamstring Stretch

Go for a walk or dance for 30 minutes

Thursday

Pull

Warm-ups: Shoulder Squeeze, Wrist Circles, Arm Swings

Standing Arm Raises

Supermans

Biceps Isometric Press

Arm Leg Raise

Friday

Rest

Saturday

Legs

Warm-ups: Leg Swings, Hip Lifts, Standing Knee Bend, Ankle Circles

Chair Squat

Standing Leg Raises

Floor Bridge

Knee Extensions

Sunday

Yoga or Rest

Cat Cow

Eagle Arms

Tree Pose

Chair Pigeon

Warrior I

Week 2

Monday
Push
Warm-ups: Arm Swings, Lateral Arm Swings, Shoulder Rolls
Incline Pushups
Dips
Wall Pushups
Plank

Tuesday
Rest

Wednesday
Pull
Warm-ups: Shoulder Squeeze, Wrist Circles, Arm Swings
Supermans
Biceps Isometric Press
Standing Arm Raises

Thursday
Cardio
Warm-ups; Leg Swings, Shoulder Rolls, Knee Bends, Seated
Hamstring Stretch
Go for a walk or dance for 30 minutes

Friday
Yoga or Rest
Reverse Arm Hold
Mountain Pose
Cobbler's Pose

Downward Facing Dog
Sphinx

Saturday
Legs
Warm-ups: Leg Swings, Lateral Leg Swings, Standing Knee Bend
Chair Squat
Standing Leg Raises
Floor Bridge
Knee Extensions

Sunday
Rest

Workout Routines with Weights

Routine 1: 6 Days Per Week

Week 1

Monday
Chest
Warm-ups: Wrist Circles, Shoulder Squeezes., Lateral Arm Swings
Floor Bench Press
Chest Fly

Tuesday
Triceps
Warm-ups: Wrist Circles, Shoulder Rolls, Neck Stretches
Overhead Triceps Extension
Dips

Wednesday
Shoulders
Warm-ups: Should Rolls, Shoulder Squeezes, Wrist Circles
Overhead Press

Bent Lateral Raise

Thursday
Cardio
Warm-ups: Wrist circles, leg swing, lateral leg swings
Weighted Walk for 20-30 minutes

Friday
Core
Warm-ups: Floor Bridge, Knee Bend, hamstring Stretch
Seated Straight Leg Lifts
Seated Oblique Stretch

Saturday
Yoga
Cat Cow
Eagle Arms
Tree Pose
Chair Pigeon
Warrior I

Sunday
Rest

Week 2

Monday
Back
Warm-ups: Shoulder Rolls, Shoulder Squeezes, Arm Swings
Bent Row
Deadlift

Tuesday

Biceps

Warm-ups: Wrist Circles, Shoulder Squeezes, Arm Swings

Dumbbell Curl

Rope Pull

Wednesday

Legs

Warm-ups: Leg Swings, Lateral Leg Swings, Knee Bend, Hip Lifts

Hip March

Calf Raises

Chair Squat

Thursday

Cardio

Warm-ups: Leg Swings, Lateral Leg Swings, Knee Bend

Farmer's Walk + Short Outdoor Walk or Dance

Friday

Core

Warm-ups: Floor Bridge, Knee Bend, hamstring Stretch

Seated Straight Leg Lifts

Seated Oblique Stretch

Saturday

Yoga

Reverse Arm Hold

Mountain Pose

Cobbler's Pose

Downward Facing Dog

Sphinx

Sunday
Rest

Routine 2: Push, Pull, Legs

Week 1

Monday
Push
Warm-ups: Arm Swings, Lateral Arm Swings, Shoulder Rolls
Overhead Press
Floor Bench
Overhead Triceps Extension

Tuesday
Rest

Wednesday
Cardio
Warm-ups: Leg Swings, Lateral Leg Swings, Knee Bend
Weighted walk 30 Minutes

Thursday
Pull
Warm-ups: Shoulder Squeeze, Wrist Circles, Arm Swings
Deadlift
Band Rows
Bicep Curl

Friday
Rest

Saturday
Legs

Warm-ups: Leg Swings, Lateral Leg Swings, Knee Bend

Hip March

Calf Raises

Chair Squat

Sunday
Yoga or Rest

Cat Cow

Eagle Arms

Tree Pose

Chair Pigeon

Warrior I

Week 2

Monday
Push

Warm-ups: Arm Swings, Lateral Arm Swings, Shoulder Rolls

Floor Bench

Chest Fly

Bent Lateral Raise

Tuesday
Rest

Wednesday
Pull

Warm-ups: Shoulder Squeeze, Wrist Circles, Arm Swings

Rope Pull

Bent Over Row

Bicep Curl

Thursday
Cardio

Warm-ups: Leg Swings, Lateral Leg Swings, Knee Bend

Farmer's Walk + Short Walk

Friday
Yoga or Rest

Reverse Arm Hold

Mountain Pose

Cobbler's Pose

Downward Facing Dog

Sphinx

Saturday
Warm-ups: Floor Bridge, Leg Swings, Lateral Leg Swings, Knee Bend

Legs

Chair Squat

Step Ups

Calf Raise

Sunday
Rest

At the Gym
Everyday

Monday
Chest

Warm-ups: Shoulder Rolls, Neck Stretches, Shoulder Squeezes, Lateral Arm Swings

Smith Machine Bench Press

Cable Press

Pushups

Tuesday
Warm-ups: Wrist Circles, Shoulder Rolls, Lateral Arm Swings
Tris
Triceps Cable Extension
Triceps Kickback

Wednesday
Shoulders
Warm-ups: Shoulder Rolls, Shoulder Squeezes., Lateral Arm Swings, Wrist Circles
Shoulder Press Machine
Bent Lateral Raises

Thursday
Cardio
Warm-ups: Leg Swings, Lateral Leg Swings, Knee Bend, Arm Swings
Elliptical Machine- 30 minutes

Friday
Core
Warm-ups: Lateral Arm Swings, Cat Cow, Leg Swings
Pallof Press
Exercise Ball Leg Balances

Saturday
Yoga
Reverse Arm Hold
Mountain Pose
Cobbler's Pose

Downward Facing Dog

Sphinx

Sunday

Rest

Monday

Back

Warm-ups: Arm Swings, Lateral Arm Swings, Shoulder Squeezes, Wrist Circles, Shoulder Rolls

Lat Pulldown

Seated Cable Row

Straight Arm Pulldown

Tuesday

Bis

Warm-ups: Arm Swings, Shoulder Squeezes, Lateral Arm Swings, Wrist Circles

Cable Curl

Dumbbell Biceps Curl

Wednesday

Legs

Warm-ups: Leg Swings, Lateral Leg Swings, Knee Bend, Hamstring Stretch, Ankle Circles

Leg Extension Machine

Leg Curl Machine

Leg Press Machine

Thursday

Cardio

Friday

Core

Warm-ups: Lateral Arm Swings, Knee Bends, Shoulder Rolls

Floor Bridge

Pallof Press

Exercise Ball Leg Balances

Saturday

Yoga

Cat Cow

Eagle Arms

Tree Pose

Chair Pigeon

Warrior I

Sunday

Rest

Push, Pull, Legs

Week 1

Monday

Push

Warm-ups: Wrist Circles, Shoulder Rolls, Shoulder Squeezes, Lateral Arm Swings

Smith Machine Bench

Shoulder Press Machine

Triceps Kickback

Arm Leg Raises

Tuesday

Rest

Wednesday
Cardio
Warm-up: Leg Swings, Knee Bend, Hamstring Stretch, Arm Swings
Elliptical Machine for 30 Minutes

Thursday
Pull
Warm-ups: Wrist Circles, Arm Swings, Shoulder Squeezes, Shoulder Rolls
Lat Pulldown
Seated Cable Row
Cable Curl
Plank

Friday
Rest

Saturday
Legs
Warm-ups: Leg Swings, Lateral Leg Swings, Knee Bend, Hamstring Stretch, Ankle Circles
Leg Extension Machine
Leg Curl Machine
Leg Press Machine
Calf Raise Machine

Sunday
Rest or Yoga
Reverse Arm Hold
Mountain Pose
Cobbler's Pose
Downward Facing Dog

Sphinx

Week 2

Monday
Push

Warm-ups: Wrist Circles, Shoulder Rolls, Shoulder Squeezes, Lateral Arm Swings

Smith Machine Bench

Shoulder Press Machine

Triceps Kickback

Plank

Tuesday
Rest

Wednesday
Pull

Warm-ups: Wrist Circles, Arm Swings, Shoulder Squeezes, Shoulder Rolls

Lat Pulldown

Seated Cable Row

Cable Curl

Exercise Ball Leg Balance

Thursday
Cardio

Warm-ups: Knee Bend, Hamstring Stretch, Leg Swings, Hip Lifts

Recumbent Bike for 30 minutes

Friday
Rest or Yoga

Cat Cow

Eagle Arms
Tree Pose
Chair Pigeon
Warrior I

Saturday

Legs
Warm-ups: Leg Swings, Lateral Leg Swings, Knee Bend, Hamstring Stretch, Ankle Circles
Leg Extension Machine
Leg Curl Machine
Leg Press Machine
Calf Raise Machine

Sunday

Rest

Conclusion

Now you have all the information you need to start and stay on your fitness journey. You can control your health and future by using the information provided in this text. Take steps to adopt a more active lifestyle, and you will feel the benefits daily.

Use your warm-ups properly before every workout to ensure you get through them without injury. They get the blood flowing and loosen you up, so exercising becomes easier. The goal of your workouts is to go through them and then come back tomorrow for another one. Consistency and putting forth a little effort every day can make all the difference.

When performing these movements, remember to focus on the task at hand. Speeding through a workout and simply moving the weights around can lead to injury, poor results, and boredom. Truly devote the time and energy to dive in and make your workouts a part of your life. Enjoy the process and feel yourself getting stronger, having more energy, sleeping better at night, and not being held back in the things you want to accomplish.

Stretching is a valuable tool that can change how you feel today and tomorrow. Take the time after workouts to stretch the muscles used to improve your workout efforts and help you get back to your day. Plan to stretch every day, if possible, regardless of your workout. Stretching helps keep you feeling young and on the path to a happier you.

Don't let exercise be a chore or a burden. Slowly work into it the way you want. You don't need to buy any equipment to get started, but when you are ready, *it will help*. Make exercising fun and a way to stay out of the doctor's office. Plan active rest days and yoga to help keep you on track. These activities will make you feel mentally and physically better as you work toward accelerating your workout program to the best level ever.

Don't forget to share your exercise journey with your friends and family. Let them know about the life-improving plans you have and all the hard work you are putting forth. Inviting some of these people to join you in your active lifestyle activities can make it even more beneficial and fun as it becomes a social venture.

Lastly, fight for your independence. The purpose of this book is to remind you of all you can do as a senior to help yourself. Make a goal and use this knowledge-packed text as the tool to achieve it. You deserve to be happy as a senior, and keeping your independence allows you to do what you want. Good luck on your journey; now, get to work!

Here's another book by Scott Hamrick that you might like

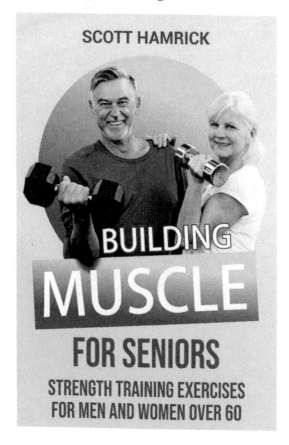

Free Bonuses from Scott Hamrick available for limited time

Hi seniors!

My name is Scott Hamrick, and first off, I want to THANK YOU for reading my book.

Now you have a chance to join my exclusive "workout for seniors" email list so you can get the ebook below for free as well as the potential to get more ebooks for seniors for free! Simply click the link below to join.

P.S. Remember that it's 100% free to join the list.

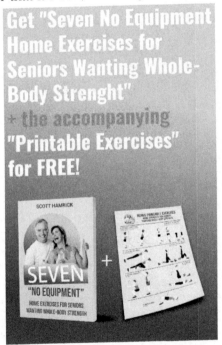

Access your free bonuses here
https://livetolearn.lpages.co/workouts-for-seniors-paperback/

Glossary of Terms

A

Abductor- 154

Anti-inflammatory 143, 144

B

Biceps 48, 50, 52, 53, 54, 59. 66, 69, 70, 71. 75

Bicep Curl 54, 58, 66

C

Chondroitin 144

Cardio

Core- The center of the body that contains the torso and abdomen and helps support and move the body.

E

Electrolytes – Essential minerals critical to human functioning that are lost through sweat. They can be replenished using exercise drinks or supplements.

Elliptical – A stationary exercise machine that requires you to stand up and use your arms and legs in constant motion as a cardiovascular activity.

Engage – To activate the muscles and hold them tight by clenching down and bracing.

Exercise Ball – A large inflatable ball capable of supporting body weight used in many balance and abdominal exercises.

Extension – Reaching or stretching a muscle, joint or limb to increase the angle between two body parts, such as extending the knee to straighten the leg.

F

Fasted – Exercising without having eaten in the last 4-8 hours beforehand to try to target fat burning.

Fed – Exercising after eating so the body has sufficient fuel to use as energy.

Flexion – Bending a muscle, limb, or joint, usually inward, such as bending an extended arm at the elbow.

G

Glucosamine – A natural substance in the body to help cushion joints that is often used as a supplement.

Glutes – The buttocks muscles used for squatting, running, and powe

H

Hamstrings – The muscles on the back of the thighs that are used for leg power, such as in deadlifting.

HIIT (High-Intensity Interval Training) – A form of exercising that uses short bursts of intense effort to help build power, improve cardio health, and burn fat.

K

Ketosis – A state in which the body relies on burning fat for energy when there are no available carbohydrates.

L

Legs – The grouping of exercises that incorporates all the movements from the waist down that use leg muscles.

M

MSM (Methylsulfonylmethane) – A dietary supplement used to help support joint health due to its anti-inflammatory properties.

N

Nutrition – The process of getting the correct and balanced foods needed for proper health and function.

O

Oblique – The flat muscle on either side of the abdominals and

Omega-3 – A healthy fatty acid found naturally but often supplemented as fish oil for its potent anti-inflammatory and cardiovascular benefits

P

Plank – An isometric exercise that helps build strength in the core and back by stabilizing the body in an elevated position.

Pull – Group of Exercises that require you to use your muscles to pull the weight towards the body or pull the body toward a fixed point.

Push – Group of exercises that require you to use your muscles to move objects away from the body or move the body away from an object.

Q

Quadriceps – The muscles on the front of the thigh used for power, such as in performing leg extensions.

R

Rep Repetition A repetition is a single performance of an exercise, such as one bicep curl.

Rest – The period between sets used to help the body recover before more work is performed.

S

Set – A set is a group of repetitions performed in a row before rest.

Smith Machine – A bench press-type machine with a barbell connected to two sliding bars for increased safety and ease of use by a single individual.

Split – A way of dividing up a weekly workout routine such as Push, Pull, and Legs.

Supplements – An add-on to the diet to help enhance nutrition or performance.

T

Triceps – The muscle on the back part of the upper arm used to push things away.

Turmeric – A natural spice and ingredient in curry often used as a supplement for its antioxidant and anti-inflammatory properties.

V

Vitamin D – An essential vitamin used to regulate the phosphate and calcium in the body, crucial to bone and joint health.

W

Warm-up – A movement used to prep an area of the body by increasing the circulation to and mobilizing the muscles.

Y

Yoga – A form of exercise that incorporates stretching, strength, balance, and breathing.